Aortic Aneurysm - Clinical Findings, Diagnostic, Treatment and Special Situations

Edited by Ana Terezinha Guillaumon and Daniel Emilio Dalledone Siqueira

Published in London, United Kingdom

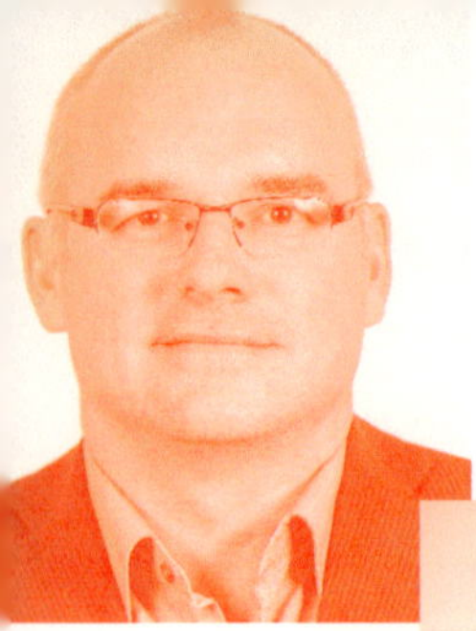
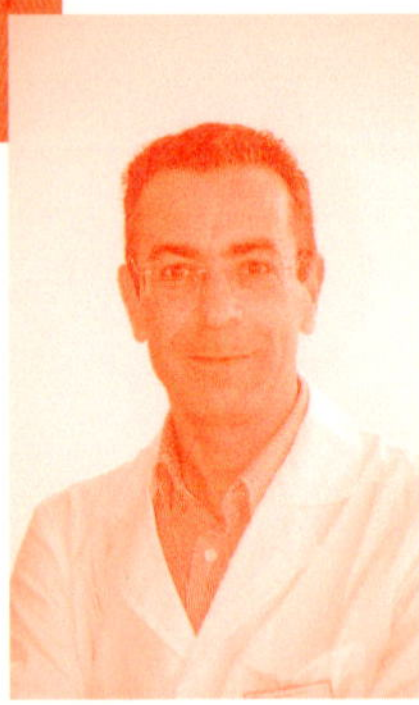
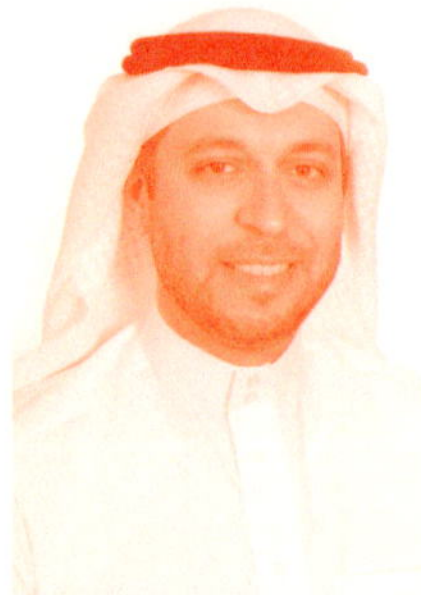
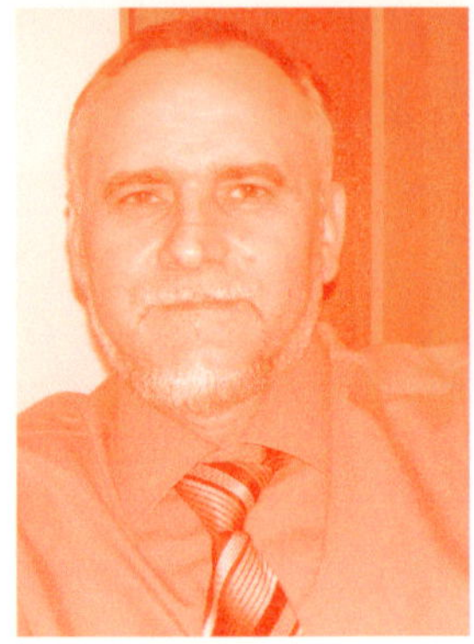
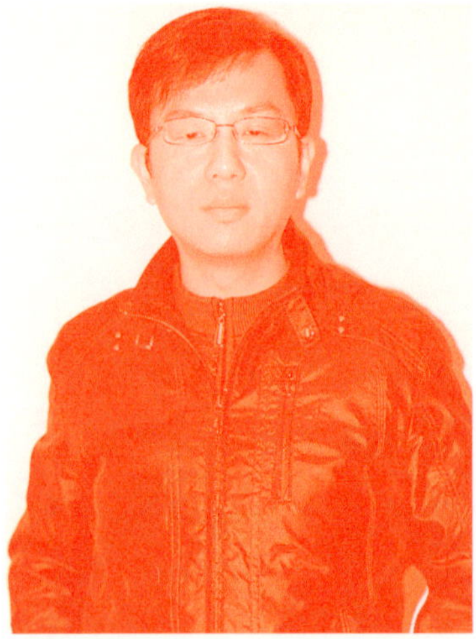
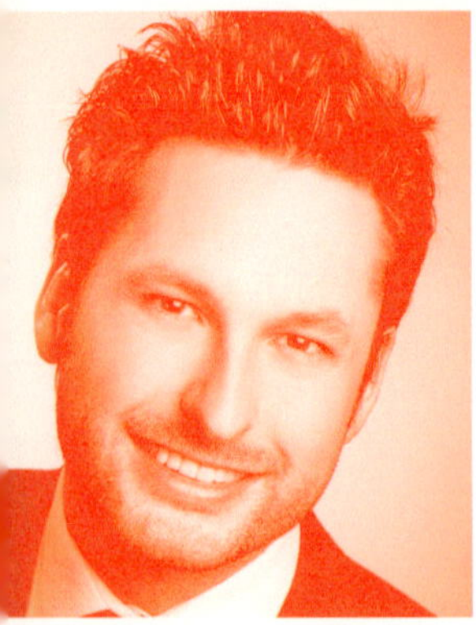
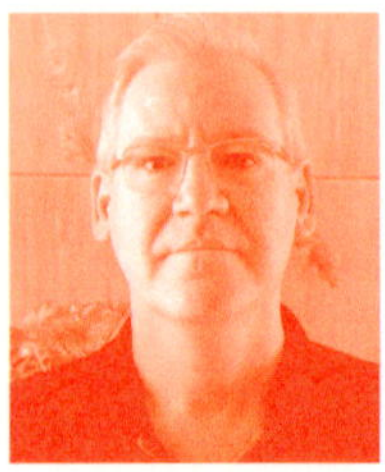

IntechOpen

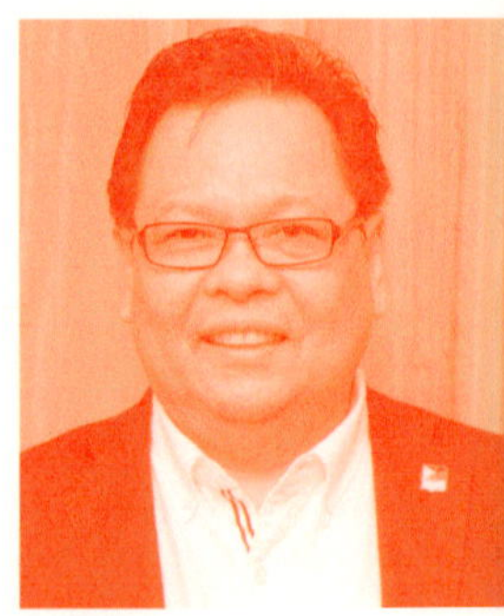
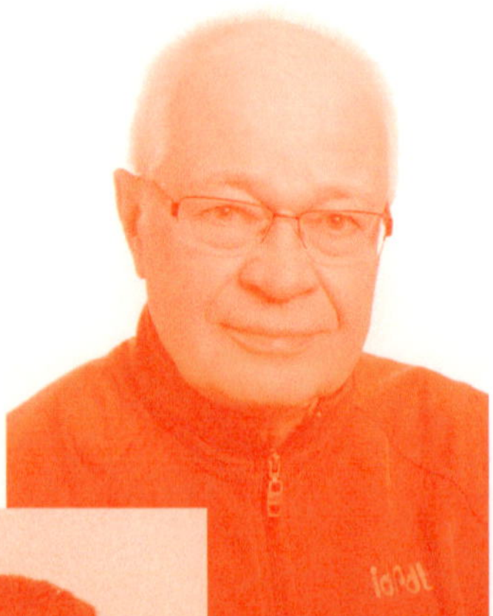
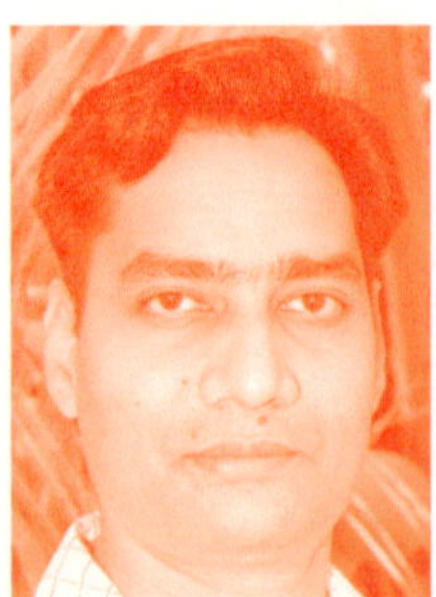
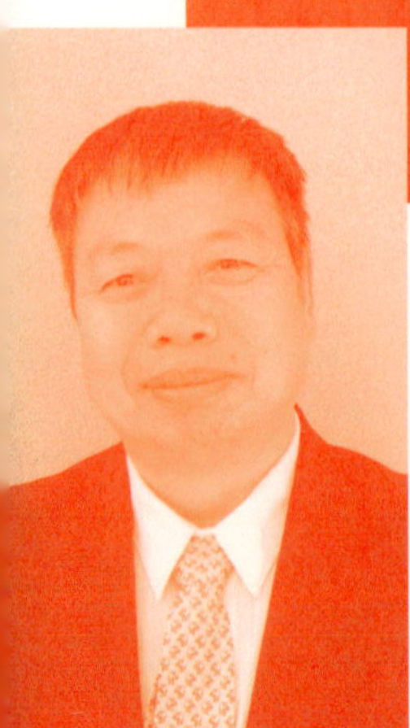
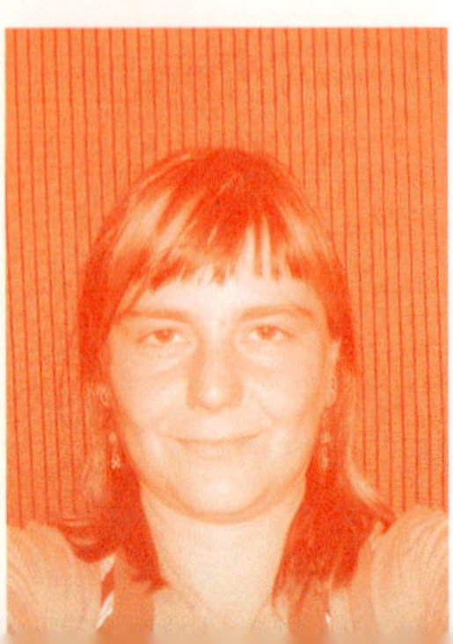
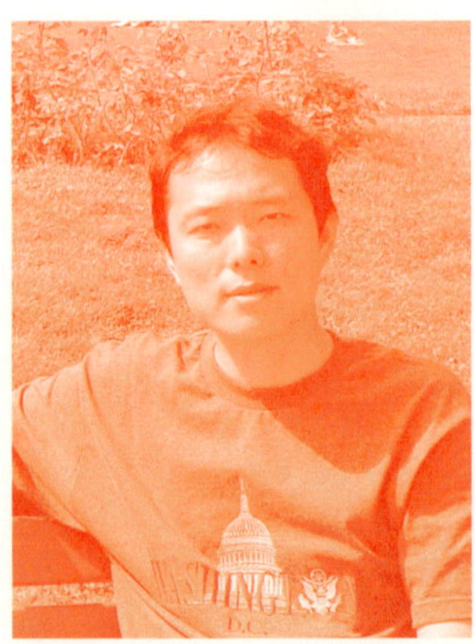

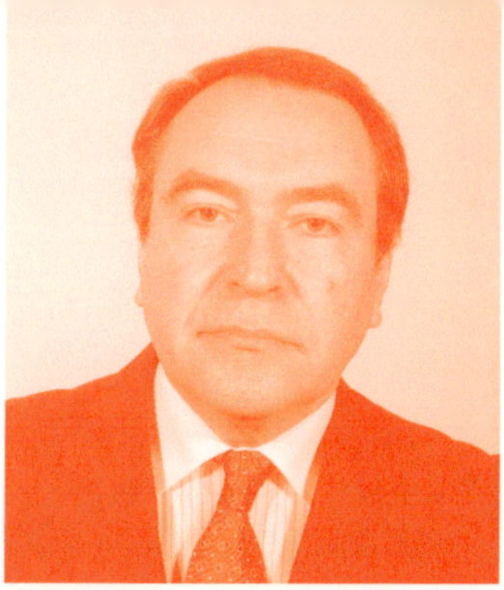
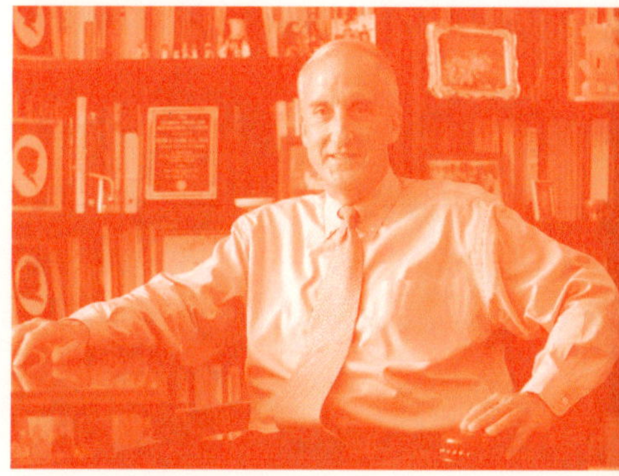
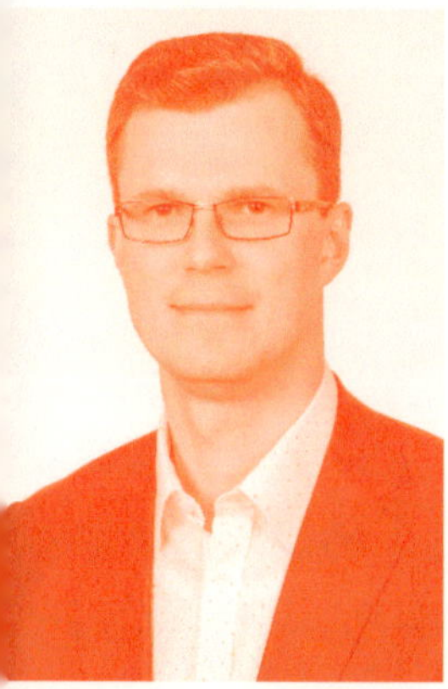
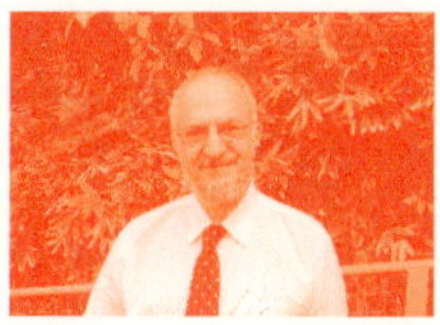
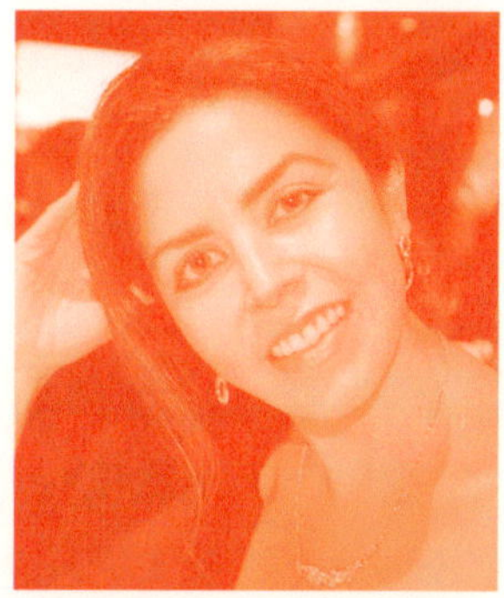

Supporting open minds since 2005

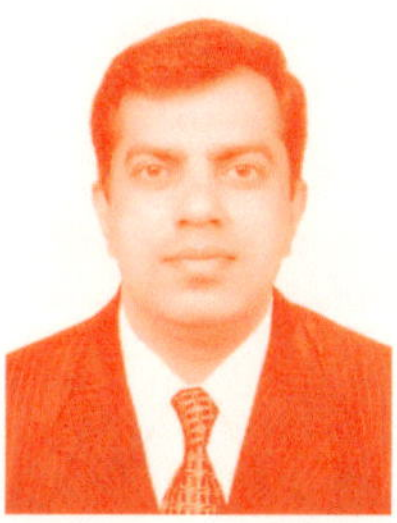
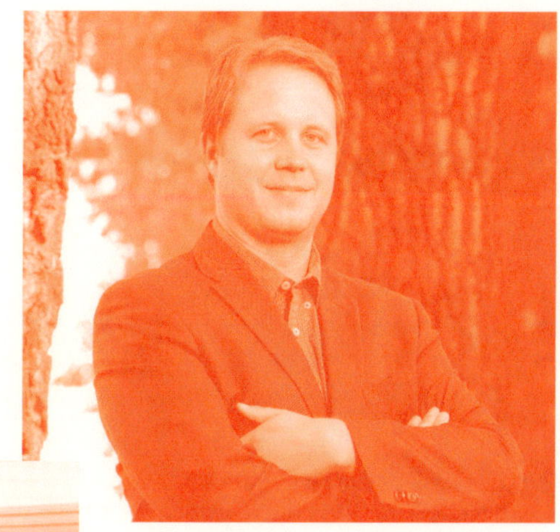
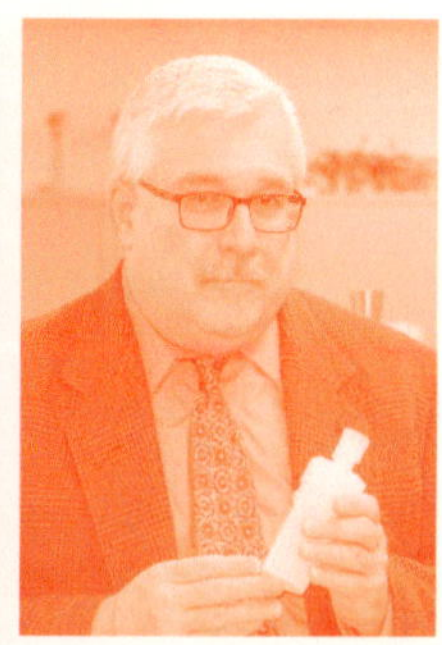
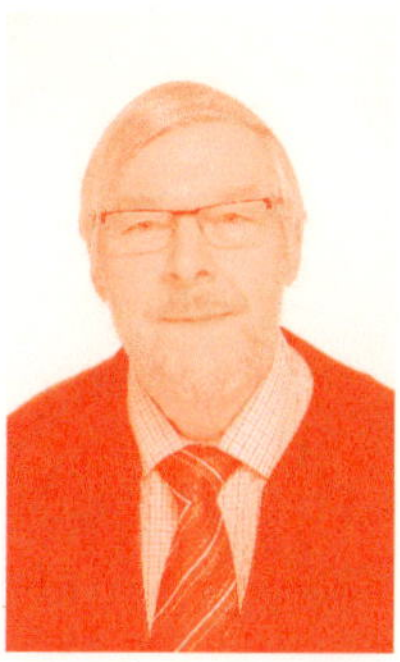
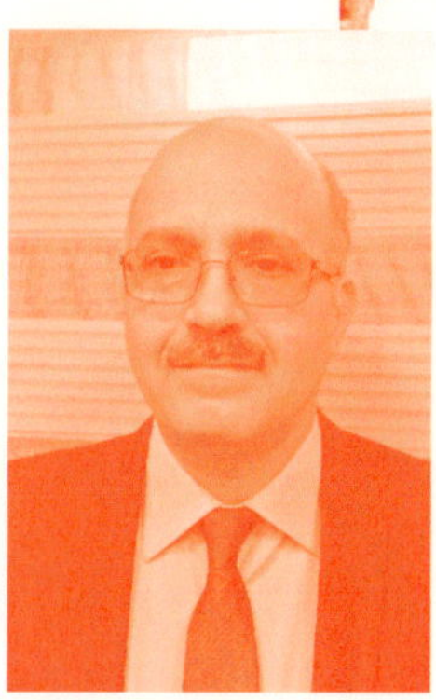
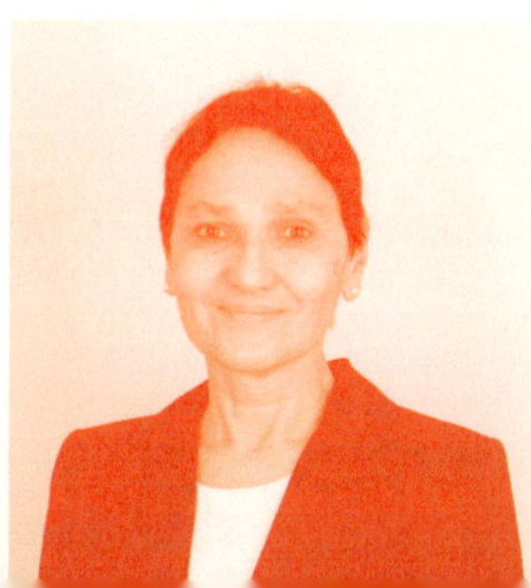
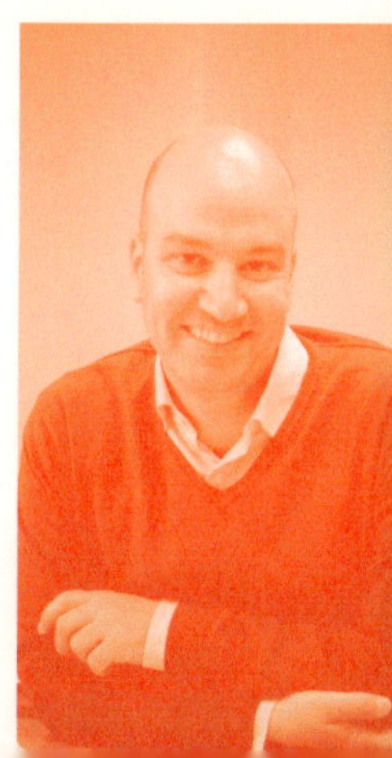

Aortic Aneurysm - Clinical Findings, Diagnostic, Treatment and Special Situations
http://dx.doi.org/10.5772/intechopen.91488
Edited by Ana Terezinha Guillaumon and Daniel Emilio Dalledone Siqueira

Contributors
Akshay Kumar, Dor Mordehay Avishay, Jennifer Chin, Marguerite Lisa Bartholomew, Enrique Ortiz Herrasti, Jorge Armando Martinez Martinez, Raúl Alberto Bacelis, Pedro Manuel Córdova, Ingrid Estrella Diaz, Kuldeep Singh, Zachary Chadnick, Luciano Izzo, Virgilio Nicolanti, Paolo Izzo, Emiliano Venditti, Sara Izzo, Daniela Messineo, Ana Terezinha Guillaumon, Daniel Emilio Dalledone Siqueira, Purnadeo Persaud, Ana Francesca Leite, Nathaniel Aoyama, Ruan Matos, Nimisha Shiwalkar, Vinit Garg, Juber Dastagir Shaikh, Roopvir Kaur, Asim Kichloo

First published in London, United Kingdom, 2021 by IntechOpen
IntechOpen is the global imprint of INTECHOPEN LIMITED, registered in England and Wales, registration number: 11086078, 5 Princes Gate Court, London, SW7 2QJ, United Kingdom
Printed in Croatia

British Library Cataloguing-in-Publication Data
A catalogue record for this book is available from the British Library

Additional hard and PDF copies can be obtained from orders@intechopen.com

Aortic Aneurysm - Clinical Findings, Diagnostic, Treatment and Special Situations
Edited by Ana Terezinha Guillaumon and Daniel Emilio Dalledone Siqueira
p. cm.
Print ISBN 978-1-83962-837-5
Online ISBN 978-1-83962-840-5
eBook (PDF) ISBN 978-1-83962-841-2

For EU product safety concerns:
IN TECH d.o.o., Prolaz Marije Krucifikse Kozulić 3, 51000 Rijeka, Croatia, info@intechopen.com or visit our website at intechopen.com.

Meet the editors

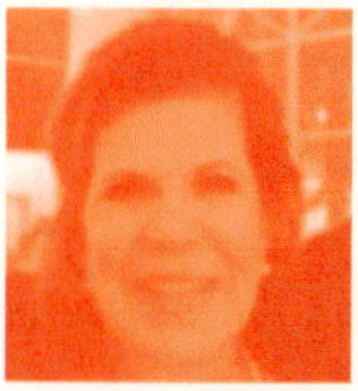

Ana Terezinha Guillaumon obtained an MD and Ph.D. in Vascular Surgery from the Surgical Science Department, School of Medical Sciences, Universidade Estadual de Campinas (UNICAMP), Campinas, Brazil. She is a full professor of Vascular Disease at the same university as well as head of the Microprocedures and Vascular Research Laboratory. She is also head of Vascular and Endovascular Surgery Hospital de Clínicas, UNICAMP. Dr. Guillaumon is a member of the Brazilian Society of Vascular Surgery (SBACV). Her areas of research interest include aortic aneurysm, ischemia and reperfusion, ischemic nephropathy, and carotid disease. She works on the development of new vascular and endovascular devices. She also serves as an editorial board member for peer-reviewed medical scientific journals.

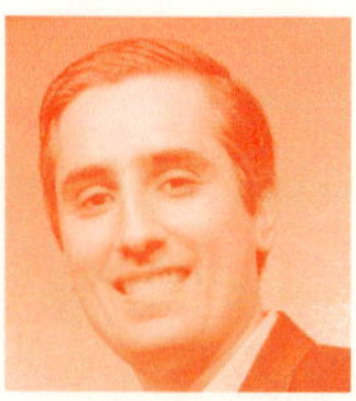

Daniel Emilio Dalledone Siqueira obtained an MD in Vascular Surgery from the Surgical Science Department, School of Medical Sciences, Universidade Estadual de Campinas (UNICAMP), Campinas, Brazil. He is currently pursuing a doctorate degree in Vascular Surgery from the same university. Dr. Siqueira is a member of the Brazilian College of Surgeons (CBC) and the Brazilian Society of Vascular Surgery (SBACV). His areas of research interest include aortic aneurysm and ischemic nephropathy. He also works on the development of new vascular and endovascular devices.

Contents

Preface

Life offers opportunities that should never be wasted, as these events bring a unique experience in carrying out a work in which we learn, teach, and expand our knowledge. This approach is essential to obtain knowledge and apply it to the care of patients with aortic aneurysm.

This work is a study of the aortic aneurysm and its various presentations. Written by eminent specialists in the field, this volume extensively covers clinical, diagnostic, and treatment findings in the aortic aneurysm. It is designed to assist in the challenging diagnosis and management of this potentially life-threatening condition. In the chapters, expert contributors share their experience and knowledge about the various aspects of aortic aneurysm disease.

For the editors, it was a privilege to participate in the edition of this book. We would like to thank the contributors and our publisher, IntechOpen.

Ana Terezinha Guillaumon
Universidade Estadual de Campinas - UNICAMP,
Brazil

Hospital de Clínicas da UNICAMP,
Brazil

Daniel Emilio Dalledone Siqueira
Universidade Estadual de Campinas - UNICAMP,
Brazil

Section 1

Aortic Aneurysm Disease

Chapter 1

Introductory Chapter: Historical Aspects and Virtues of the Aortic Surgeon

Ana Terezinha Guillaumon and Daniel Emilio Dalledone Siqueira

1. Introduction

The history and description of abdominal aortic aneurysms is as old as mankind. The earliest accounts date back to the Hearst Papyrus, an integral part of the Eber Papyrus of ancient Egypt, circa 1500 BC. There is also mention of this disease in the Sushruta Samhita manuscript from 800 to 600 BC, written by Sushruta, founder of Ayurvedic medicine [1–3]. Several authors continued describing specific aspects of aortic aneurysm disease, such as Galen and Antyllus. At that time, there was no treatment described for aortic aneurysm repair [4].

However, the evolution of the treatment of abdominal aortic aneurysms only occurred in 1817, when Cooper performed the first aortic ligation for the treatment of a ruptured external iliac artery aneurysm [3]. The patient died four hours after the procedure. It was only in 1923 that the first successful surgical treatment for the treatment of arterial aneurysm occurred, being responsible for the development of the endoaneurysmorrhaphy technique [5]. Several surgeons worked hard, in the 19th and 20th centuries, to develop safe surgical treatment methods with low mortality. Nissen performed the surgical treatment of an abdominal aortic aneurysm in Albert Einstein by wrapping him in cellophane [6, 7]. This surgery allowed Einstein to live more 7 years.

Alexis Carrel contributed significantly to vascular surgery. He developed the techniques of vascular anastomosis, allowing new perspectives in the treatment of abdominal aortic aneurysms [1–3]. In 1952, Arthur Vorhees performed the repair of a ruptured aortic aneurysm with a synthetic graft, applying vascular anastomosis techniques, marking the beginning of the golden age of aortic surgery [8].

Great surgeons such as Ernest Stanley Crawford, Michael Ellis DeBakey and Denton Arthur Cooley improved vascular surgical techniques, introducing sequential clamping methods, with shorter ischemia times [9]. As a result, they obtained fantastic results in open abdominal aortic surgery.

The research and improvements in abdominal aortic surgery continued over the years, allowing new technical options to be developed. Juan Carlos Parodi 1976 began the study of grafts for endovascular use. However, it was only in 1990 that Parodi performed the first successful endovascular surgery in humans [10].

Aortic aneurysm disease continues to be the source of numerous studies. New perspectives in identifying etiology, pathophysiology, diagnosis and treatment should be encouraged. Surgical treatment has advanced significantly in recent years with less invasive techniques and lower morbidity and mortality.

This book aims to provide an objective technical and scientific approach to abdominal aortic aneurysm disease. In addition to the aspects inherent to technical knowledge of aortic aneurysmal disease for successful treatment, the surgeon must have the skills and virtues.

IntechOpen

2. The virtues of the aorta surgeon

The surgeon, especially those who approach the aorta, sometimes faces situations that are almost impossible to correct and it is at this moment that we feel the limit of our performance. There is the treatment for all patients, but it depends on the medical technical decision associated with the patient's care. Therefore, the clear and objective explanation to the patient, the "steps" to be followed, is a joint and fundamental action for the success of the treatment, whatever it may be. Thus, a doctor-patient relationship is built, whose trust implements the treatment actions.

The surgeon does his/her work far beyond the purely technical aspects. Well, the construction of a career as a surgeon cannot be only technical but based on moral aspects and humanism. We will discuss the four virtues that must be developed and are essential to a good surgeon.

The first virtue is courage, it represents the beginning and is most admired for its ability to overcome fear. The fear of approaching the largest vessel in the human body, which is the aorta, is responsible for bringing life to all tissues and organs. This virtue is not a spectacle and is never seen as a success. Courage is a virtue that is present in the lives of heroes, who believe in their principles: it serves to think well, to advance or retreat, especially in operative approaches.

The second virtue is humility, a singular virtue because the surgeon's self-works. It makes the surgeon not proud of his/her technical preparation and surgical results. This virtue awakens the surgeon to the awareness of the impotence of imitating God, without being so. It also allows the surgeon to be clear about reality and possible difficulties.

The third virtue is prudence, it is the exercise of the superego leading the professional to do and choose what is absolutely necessary. Avoiding acts opposite to necessary in the treatment of the patient. Prudence has as its principle the condition of fidelity between technique and absolute character. It is a structural part of medical ethics.

The fourth virtue is simplicity, it is the lightest of virtues. This one is unquestionable, it is just real. Simplicity summarizes existence. It is virtue linked to intelligence, it turns complex actions into simple actions.

We believe that the union between technical and scientific knowledge associated with the virtues allows for greater humanism in the doctor-patient relationship.

Author details

Ana Terezinha Guillaumon[1,2]* and Daniel Emilio Dalledone Siqueira[2]

1 Hospital de Clínicas da Unicamp, São Paulo, Brazil

2 Universidade Estadual de Campinas, São Paulo, Brazil

*Address all correspondence to: atguillaumon@gmail.com

References

[1] Nevitt MP, Ballard DJ, Hallett JW Jr. Prognosis of abdominal aortic aneurysms. A population-based study. The New England Journal of Medicine. 1989; **321**(15):1009-1014

[2] Friedman SG. A History of Vascular Surgery. New York: Futura Publishing Company; 1989

[3] Suy R. The varying morphology and aetiology of the arterial aneurysm. A historical review. Acta Chirurgica Belgica. 2006;**106**(3):354-360

[4] Berge C, Haug ES, Romundstad PR, Lange C, Myhre HO. Infrarenal abdominal aortic aneurysm repair: Time-trends during a 20-year period. World Journal of Surgery. 2007;**31**(8): 1682-1686

[5] Cordell AR. A lasting legacy: The life and work of Rudolph Matas. Journal of Vascular Surgery. 1985;**2**(4):613-619

[6] Cohen JR, Graver LM. The ruptured abdominal aortic aneurysm of Albert Einstein. Surgery, Gynecology & Obstetrics. 1990;**170**(5):455-458

[7] Lytton DG, Resuhr LM. Galen on abnormal swellings. Journal of the History of Medicine and Allied Sciences. 1978;**33**(4):531-549

[8] Voorhees AB Jr. The development of arterial prostheses: A personal view. Archives of Surgery. 1985;**120**(3):289-295

[9] Livesay JJ, Messner GN, Vaughn WK. Milestones in the treatment of aortic aneurysm: Denton A. Cooley, MD, and the Texas Heart Institute. Texas Heart Institute Journal. 2005;**32**(2):130-134

[10] Thompson JE. Early history of aortic surgery. Journal of Vascular Surgery. 1998;**28**(4):746-752

Chapter 2

Alternative Techniques for Treatment of Thoracic Aneurysms without Ideal Anatomy

Jorge Armando Martinez, Enrique Ortiz Herrasti, Raúl Alberto Bacelis, Pedro Manuel Córdova and Ingrid Estrella Diaz

Abstract

The combination of open surgery and thoracic endovascular repair [TEVAR] are considered hybrid procedures, they are used today to solve the different pathologies of the thoracic aorta, these procedures are presented as a therapeutic alternative for those patients who are not candidates for a procedure conventional surgical procedure, either because they are considered "high risk" patients, due to their pathological history, or in those patients who present a complex anatomy that makes it difficult to complete the repair with endovascular therapies in its entirety. To familiarize ourselves with these therapies, we consider it important to classify them by anatomical segments according to the Ishimaru classification to facilitate their understanding.

Keywords: thoracic aorta, aneurysm, hybrid, endovascular, bypass, endovascular, debranching

1. Introduction

Managing thoracic aortic aneurysms involving the aortic arch poses a surgical challenge. Open surgery it is the gold standard procedure that uses a medium sternotomy and cardiopulmonary bypass [CPB] and hypothermic circulatory arrest is associated with significant morbidity and mortality which causes patients at "high risk" determined by the American Society of Anesthesiologists [ASA] do not be candidates for this kind of repair. Endovascular therapy has revolutionized the treatment of complex chest aortic disease, but supra-aortic arch anatomy represents a more complex challenge for endovascular therapy, although new techniques have resulted such as fenestrated and branched stents these are still in the experimental stage. Treatment hybrid is a combination of debranching procedures of the branches of the supra-aortic arch with endovascular repair of the chest aorta, it is a good alternative in patients with difficult anatomy and high-risk, obtain technical satisfaction in most cases. Hybrid therapy has several studies with promising results but has not been validated as an option of treatment today.

2. Classification of techniques alternative for treatment of thoracic aneurysms involving the aortic arch

Volodos team performed the first hybrid aortic arch repair in 1991. Since then, it has grown enormously by the development of these alternative therapies to conventional open surgery [1].

Indications for repair of thoracic aortic aneurysms are mostly from aneurysm degeneration greater than 5.5 cm in 54% al 63% and secondly dissections by 22% al 43% emergency procedures are performed in up to 20% of cases.

Patients undergoing hybrid repair mention among their history chronic obstructive pulmonary disease secondary to smoking and ischemic cardiac history in 12%, ischemic brain events at 10%, and 16% of patients have the antecedent of a repair of an abdominal aortic aneurysm [2, 3].

The reported complication rates for thoracic aortic interventions are estimated to be 36% in procedures performed entirely with endovascular therapy using fenestrated/branched endografts. When hybrid procedures are performed, the complication rate is 33%, and 50% for open surgery [4].

Regarding the complications reported after hybrid therapies, we found that patients present endoleaks with rates between 9% and 22% of cases, most endoleaks are type 1 and are resolved in the vast majority of cases with the placement of a proximal prosthesis or extension, stroke is reported in 7% to 14% of patients, mainly related to the posterior circulation, probably related to the occlusion of the left subclavian artery that is performed in a programmed way in the majority of cases, paraplegia in 0.5% to 6% with response to cerebrospinal fluid drainage in one third of patients, this drainage is recommended in patients with extensive aortic disease or after placing an endoprosthesis with an extension greater than 15 cm in length. The descending aorta, retrograde aortic dissection in 4.1%, this occurs more frequently in hybrid therapies in which covered stents parallel to the aortic are used, and graft bypass occlusion 4% and cardiopulmonary complications 14%. [5–8].

The technical satisfaction of hybrid procedures is estimated between 69% and 100% with an average of 87% of the cases, with a conversion to open surgery of 3% for the repair of any complication. Rate survival to 12-month after the procedure is 78%, and the 3-year follow-up is reported at 73% [5, 6, 8].

Regarding the surgical approaches used to access the carotid arteries, a longitudinal or transverse incision in the neck is used more frequently, for the left subclavian artery a horizontal infraclavicular or supraclavicular incision is used, the latter being the most used, some patients require of a median sternotomy to approach a healthy segment of the ascending aorta and place a graft with 2 or 3 branches in it to completely reimplant the aortic arch. Hybrid repair offers good short-term results, but more long-term follow-up studies of bypass results and permeability are needed in these patients. Follow-up studies of complex thoracic aneurysms with hybrid procedures are mostly retrospective some with 36-month follow-up [1, 4].

The debranching procedures are divided into complete procedures when the debranching corresponds to zone 0 of the Ishimaru classification with which the three main branches of the aortic arch are reconstructed, the partial procedures are those that correspond to the zone 1 and 2 of Ishimaru, in zone 1 the left carotid artery and the left subclavian artery are reconstructed and in zone 2 the left subclavian artery only [9].

2.1 Zone 0

Zone 0 corresponds to the ascending aorta and the origin of the innominate artery. Hybrid reconstructions in this area can be subdivided into two types:

2.1.1 Type 1

Type 1 is used when a segment of the ascending aorta is healthy, this repair consists of the reimplantation of the aortic arch vessels, using a 2 or 3-branch dacron graft that is anastomosed to a healthy ascending aorta segment above of the tubular sinus junction. The left subclavian artery is the first to anastomosed followed by the left carotid artery and later the brachiocephalic trunk, in the case that the left subclavian artery is not accessible by a sternotomy, a left carotid artery bypass is performed to the left subclavian artery through a supraclavicular incision. This procedure can be performed with a cardiopulmonary pump or by lateral clamping of a segment of the aorta, using a mean time of 193 ± 58 minutes and a mean clamping time of 44 ± 27 minutes. When using a 2-limb graft, the need to bypass the left carotid artery to the left subclavian artery should be evaluated at the time of surgery or later **Figure 1** [1, 8, 10, 11].

2.1.2 Type 2

This type of repair is performed in those patients with extensive disease of the ascending aorta in which there is no healthy segment to perform a type 1 repair, or when the ascending aorta that corresponds to the proximal landing zone of the endoprosthesis is greater than 3.7 cm since this diameter is associated with a greater risk of type A dissection. This repair consists of the substitution of the ascending aorta with a dacron graft and a 2 or 3-branch dacron graft is anastomosed on this graft. This repair requires the use of a cardiopulmonary pump and sometimes a

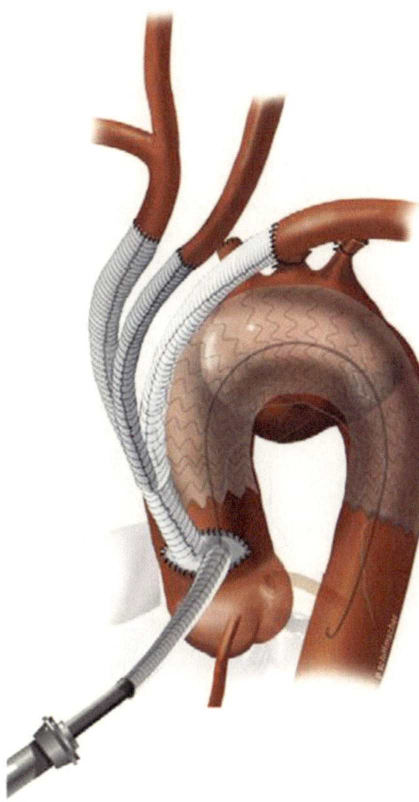

Figure 1.
Debranching zone 0 type 1, using a 3 branch dacron graft, the endoprosthesis covering the three main branches of the aortic arch.

short period of circulatory arrest with a mean time of 259 ± 54 minutes with clamping time of 121 ± 63 minutes of circulatory arrest **Figure 2** [1, 8, 10].

The following are recommendations when performing aortic arch reconstruction:

1. Mean arterial pressure of 80-100 mmHg during anastomosis of the arteries supplying the head.

2. Have prefabricated grafts of 2, 3 or 4 branches.

3. Start the reconstruction with the anastomosis on the anterolateral aspect of the ascending aorta.

4. During the anterior anastomosis maintain a mean arterial pressure of 50-60 mmHg.

5. Continue with the revascularization from distal to proximal starting with the left subclavian artery, followed by the left common carotid artery and finally the brachiocephalic trunk.

6. During the previous anastomosis, maintain a mean arterial pressure between 80-100 mmHg.

7. When the left subclavian artery is not accessible through the median sternotomy, a carotid-subclavian bypass is performed through a supraclavicular incision at the same time or later.

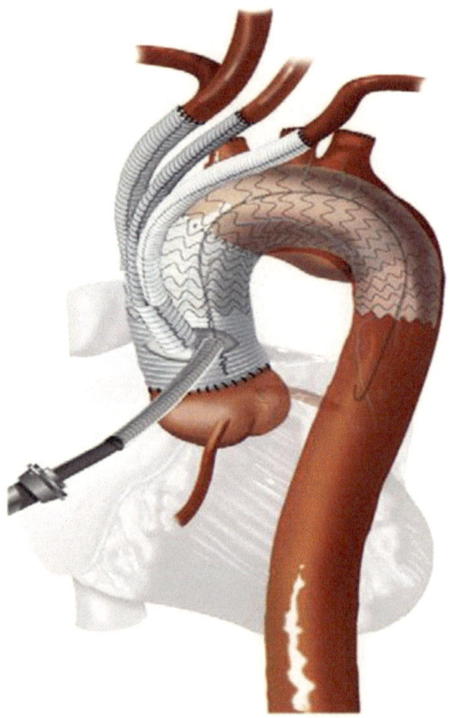

Figure 2.
Debranching zone 0 type 2, using a 3 branch dacron graft, the substitution of the ascending aorta with a dacron graft and endoprosthesis covering the three main branches of the aortic arch.

In general, the 30-day in-hospital mortality reported for these procedures is 8% to 14%, with the highest mortality for type 2 procedures, a neurological deficit of 7% to 14%, and kidney failure requiring hemodialysis in 3%. Atrial fibrillation is reported in up to 42% of these patients, the reported survival is 71%, 60%, and 48% at 12 months, 3, and 5 years, respectively [1, 8, 11].

2.2 Zone 1

Zone 1 corresponds to the area of the ascending aorta between the brachycephalic trunk and the left common carotid artery. Repair of the left subclavian artery may or may not be necessary, depending on the clinical context, this repair is performed in up to 70% of cases, so repair is recommended whenever possible. The debranching of zone 1 is a partial procedure and is subdivided into three types:

2.2.1 Type 1

Sequential bypass from right carotid to left carotid and left subclavian artery is carried out by performing a sequential bypass that is: An anastomosis of the right carotid artery to the left carotid artery and from this a bypass to the left subclavian artery, so this procedure can be completed without the need for extracorporeal circulation, median sternotomy, or thoracotomy (**Figure 3**).

2.2.2 Type 2

Double arterial transposition this is to perform an anastomosis first from the left carotid artery to the right carotid artery or the brachiocephalic trunk followed

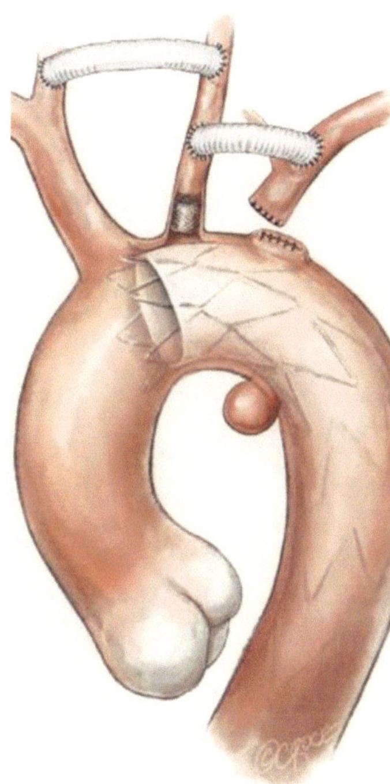

Figure 3.
Debranching zone 1 type 1, using bypass sequential bypass from right carotid to left carotid and left subclavian artery. Note closure of the left carotid artery lumen and ligation of the left subclavian artery, with a endoprosthesis covering two branches of the aortic arch.

by an anastomosis between the left subclavian artery to the left carotid artery. A single transposition of the left carotid artery to the right carotid artery can also be performed followed by a left carotid artery bypass to the left subclavian artery using a graft [1, 8] (**Figure 4**).

2.2.3 Type 3

Bypass with graft of the right carotid artery to the left subclavian artery, then the insertion of the left carotid artery over the graft is performed [6].

There are no studies comparing the three types of hybrid revascularization for zone 1 (**Figure 5**).

2.3 Zone 2

The debranching of zone 2 is a partial procedure too.

Many patients with thoracic aortic disease have extension of the disease to the left subclavian artery, so it may need to be covered between 40% and 50% to achieve a seal and adequate proximal fixation. In general, after TEVAR the rates of neurological complications are up to 15%, the etiology is related to athero-embolization and decreased flow of the left vertebral artery [7, 10, 12]. Some authors suggest that the coverage of the left subclavian artery is associated with an increase in neurological complications related to the reduction of the flow of the posterior circulation, while others report that revascularizing the left subclavian artery does not offer any benefit, on the contrary, it increases the surgical time and the risk of complications, especially in emergency surgeries such as ruptured aortic aneurysm [10, 12].

In 2010 the published guidelines of the Society for Vascular Surgery [SVS] and in 2017 the guidelines of the European Society for Vascular Surgery [ESVS] recommend early revascularization of the left subclavian artery to reduce the

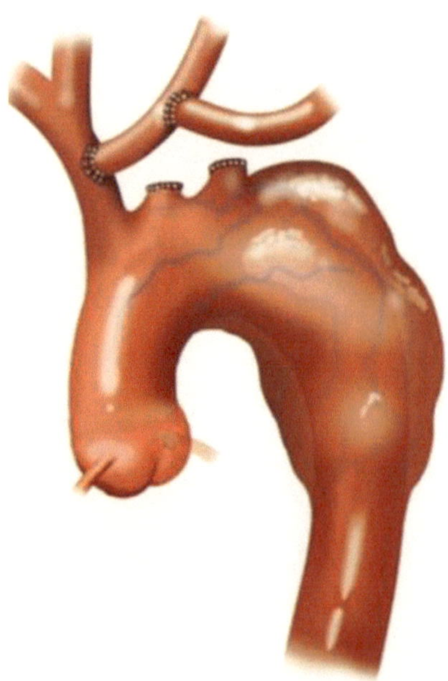

Figure 4.
Debranching zone 1 type 2, using double arterial transposition. Note closure of the lumen of the left carotid artery and the left subclavian artery with a suture line.

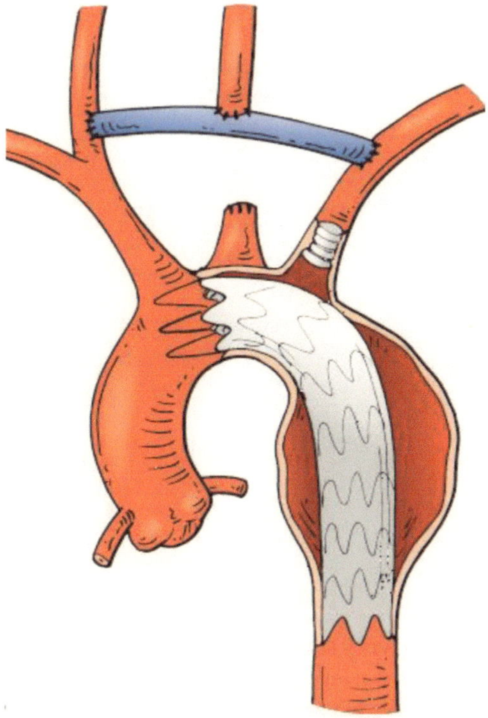

Figure 5.
Debranching zone 1 type 3, using bypass with graft. Note closure of the lumen of the left subclavian artery whit coils and the left carotid artery with a suture line, with a endoprosthesis covering two branches of the aortic arch.

risk of neurological complications, but this recommendation is based on low-quality evidence [13, 14].

In the meta-analysis published in 2016 [15], which compared retrospective studies, they found a stroke rate of 2.2% to 5.8% for patients with left subclavian artery revascularization and from 7.8% to 9.1% In those who did not revascularize, with respect to spinal cord ischemia, a rate of 2.7% was reported for those patients with revascularization and 4.3% for those patients without revascularization of the left subclavian artery, without statistical significance for these results, but with a trend in favor of revascularization of the left subclavian artery.

Factors related to stroke and spinal ischemia include the duration of the procedure, the degree of underlying aortic disease, device navigation and release, the number of prostheses used in aortic repair, occlusion below T10, insufficiency renal and female sex [15–18]. Mortality from revascularization and non-revascularization of the left subclavian artery in hybrid procedures is similar, 3.1% to 4.3% respectively.

There is no significant difference in the effectiveness between open revascularization surgery techniques (left carotid-subclavian shunt or subclavian carotid transposition), finding 100% patency in the two techniques. Open revascularization is not without complications such as lymphatic leakage, vocal cord paralysis in 5% to 13%, and phrenic nerve injury in 4.4% of cases [10, 19].

In recent years, a tendency has been observed to revascularize the left subclavian artery with endovascular techniques; Some studies suggest that these revascularization techniques present similar results to open surgery, whether it is the transposition of the left subclavian artery to the left carotid artery or the bypass of the left carotid artery to the left subclavian artery, in selected patients, such as:

Preoperative	Intraoperative	Postoperative
• Bypass in the internal mammary artery (IMA).	• Loss of left radial pulse after device deployment.	• Clinical symptoms of vertebrobasilar insufficiency (ataxia, blurred vision, dizziness).
• Left vertebral artery (LVA) direct branch of the aortic arch.		• Claudication of the left arm.
• Access for hemodialysis in the left thoracic limb (LTL).		
• Dominant left vertebral artery.		
• Protection of the spinal cord.		
• Extensive coverage of the aorta		

Table 1.
Indications for revascularization of the left subclavian artery. This table considers three moments in which we can perform a surgery.

patients with severe obesity, very short and stiff necks, previous neck surgeries. For endovascular therapy of the left subclavian artery to be performed, anatomical aspects should be considered such as: a distance greater than 40 mm between the left vertebral artery and the subclavian artery left, an angle less than 75 degrees to the aortic arch of the left subclavian artery [3, 17].

Most of these studies do not describe anatomical details that determine the result, and the evidence is based on a small number of clinical cases with short-term follow-up of [17, 18]. Therefore, the surgeon must individualize the best therapeutic option for each patient based on the least morbidity and the longest possible duration.

The indications for elective revascularization of the ASI can be summarized in **Table 1** [16, 18].

3. Conclusion

There are no data from randomized controlled trials comparing conventional therapy with hybrid procedures for the treatment of aortic arch pathology; some studies comparing the results between open surgery and hybrid therapies show a statistically significant findings found in recent studies a reduction in mortality. However, hybrid procedures are an alternative for those patients with high surgical risk who cannot tolerate open repair or complex anatomy for endovascular therapy.

Conflicts of interest

The authors have no conflicts of interest to declare.

Thanks

To my teachers and my wife, Martha Julia, for their support and dedication.

Recognitions

The authors did not receive financial support for the research, authorship and/or publication of this chapter.

Author details

Jorge Armando Martinez*, Enrique Ortiz Herrasti, Raúl Alberto Bacelis, Pedro Manuel Córdova and Ingrid Estrella Diaz
Regional Hospital of High Specialty of the Yucatan Peninsula, Mérida City, Mexico

*Address all correspondence to: sturiyamni@gmail.com

References

[1] Preventza O, Garcia A, Cooley DA, et al. Total aortic arch replacement: A comparative study of zone 0 hybrid arch exclusion versus traditional open repair Read at the 95th Annual Meeting of the American Association for Thoracic Surgery, Seattle, Washington, April 25-29, 2015. J Thorac Cardiovasc Surg. 2015;150(6):1591-1600. doi:10.1016/j.jtcvs.2015.08.117

[2] Nashef SAM, Roques F, Sharples LD, et al. Euroscore II. Eur J Cardio-thoracic Surg. 2012;41(4):734-745. doi:10.1093/ejcts/ezs043

[3] Iba Y, Minatoya K, Matsuda H, et al. How should aortic arch aneurysms be treated in the endovascular aortic repair era? A risk-adjusted comparison between open and hybrid arch repair using propensity score-matching analysis. Eur J Cardio-thoracic Surg. 2014;46(1):32-39. doi:10.1093/ejcts/ezt615

[4] D'Oria M, Kärkkäinen JM, Tenorio ER, et al. Perioperative Outcomes of Carotid–Subclavian Bypass or Transposition versus Endovascular Techniques for Left Subclavian Artery Revascularization during Nontraumatic Zone 2 Thoracic Endovascular Aortic Repair in the Vascular Quality Initiative. Ann Vasc Surg. 2020;69:17-26. doi:10.1016/j.avsg.2020.05.062

[5] Lotfi S, Clough RE, Ali T, et al. Hybrid repair of complex thoracic aortic arch pathology: Long-term outcomes of extra-anatomic bypass grafting of the supra-aortic trunk. Cardiovasc Intervent Radiol. 2013;36(1):46-55. doi:10.1007/s00270-012-0383-3

[6] Antoniou GA, El Sakka K, Hamady M, Wolfe JHN. Hybrid Treatment of Complex Aortic Arch Disease with Supra-aortic Debranching and Endovascular Stent Graft Repair. Eur J Vasc Endovasc Surg. 2010;39(6):683-690. doi:10.1016/j.ejvs.2010.02.002

[7] M. Christopher AMLS. 乳鼠心肌提取 HHS Public Access. Physiol Behav. 2016;176(1):100-106. doi:10.1016/j.jamcollsurg.2015.02.028.Outcomes

[8] Chakos A, Jbara D, Yan TD, Tian DH. Long-term survival and related outcomes for hybrid versus traditional arch repair-A meta-analysis. Ann Cardiothorac Surg. 2018;7(3):319-327. doi:10.21037/acs.2018.05.07

[9] Ishimaru S. Endografting of the aortic arch. J Endovasc Ther. 2004;11(SUPPL. 2):6-7. doi:10.1583/04-1407.1

[10] Bavaria J, Vallabhajosyula P, Moeller P, Szeto W, Desai N, Pochettino A. Hybrid approaches in the treatment of aortic arch aneurysms: Postoperative and midterm outcomes. J Thorac Cardiovasc Surg. 2013;145(3 SUPPL.):85-90. doi:10.1016/j.jtcvs.2012.11.044

[11] Tian DH, Wan B, Di Eusanio M, Black D, Yan TD. A systematic review and meta-analysis on the safety and efficacy of the frozen elephant trunk technique in aortic arch surgery. Ann Cardiothorac Surg. 2013;2(5):581-591. doi:10.3978/j.issn.2225-319X.2013.09.07

[12] Patterson BO, Holt PJ, Nienaber C, Fairman RM, Heijmen RH, Thompson MM. Management of the left subclavian artery and neurologic complications after thoracic endovascular aortic repair. J Vasc Surg. 2010;60(6):1491-1498.e1. doi:10.1016/j.jvs.2014.08.114

[13] Matsumura JS, Lee WA, Mitchell RS, Farber MA, Murad MH, Lumsden AB, et al. The Society for Vascular Surgery Practice Guidelines: Management of

the left subclavian artery with thoracic endovascular aortic repair. J Vasc Surg [Internet]. 2009;50(5):1155-8. Available from: http://dx.doi.org/10.1016/j.jvs.2009.08.090

[14] Writing Committee, Riambau V, Böckler D, Brunkwall J, Cao P, Chiesa R, et al. Editor's Choice – Management of Descending Thoracic Aorta Diseases: Clinical Practice Guidelines of the European Society for Vascular Surgery (ESVS). Eur J Vasc Endovasc Surg [Internet]. 2017;53(1):4-52. Available from: http://dx.doi.org/10.1016/j.ejvs.2016.06.005

[15] Piffaretti G, Pratesi G, Gelpi G, Galli M, Criado FJ, Antonello M, et al. Comparison of Two Different Techniques for Isolated Left Subclavian Artery Revascularization During Thoracic Endovascular Aortic Repair in Zone 2. J Endovasc Ther. 2018;25(6):740-9. DOI: 10.1177/1526602818802581

[16] Sobocinski J, Patterson BO, Karthikesalingam A, Thompson MM. The Effect of Left Subclavian Artery Coverage in Thoracic Endovascular Aortic Repair. Ann Thorac Surg [Internet]. 2016;101(2):810-7. Available from: http://dx.doi.org/10.1016/j.athoracsur.2015.08.069

[17] Bradshaw RJ, Ahanchi SS, Powell O, Larion S, Brandt C, Soult MC, et al. Left subclavian artery revascularization in zone 2 thoracic endovascular aortic repair is associated with lower stroke risk across all aortic diseases. J Vasc Surg [Internet]. 2010;1-10. Available from: http://dx.doi.org/10.1016/j.jvs.2016.10.111

[18] Hajibandeh S, Hajibandeh S, Antoniou SA, Torella F, Antoniou GA. Meta-analysis of Left Subclavian Artery Coverage With and Without Revascularization in Thoracic Endovascular Aortic Repair. 2016; DOI 10.1177/152660281665141

[19] Martínez-Martínez J, Ortiz-Herrasti E, Martínez-Cachón JE, Lecuona-Huet NE, Farro-Moreno A, Moreno-Vargas HC. Manejo híbrido de aneurisma de aorta torácica descendente. Rev Mex Angiol. 2019;47(1):47-51. ISSN: 00377740

Chapter 3

Aortic Aneurysm: A Surgical Point of View

Luciano Izzo, Daniela Messineo, Emiliano Venditti, Virgilio Nicolanti, Sara Izzo and Paolo Izzo

Abstract

Aortic aneurysms are of different types as different ones are the types of treatment available to us. Following the advent of endovascular surgery, perioperative mortality has been significantly reduced, but open surgery remains the first choice under some occurrences. The purpose of this chapter is to try to clarify the dichotomy between open and endovascular aortic aneurysms in the several types of aortic aneurysms, highlighting the indications and complications to guide to the best therapeutic choice.

Keywords: EVAR, TEVAR, open, endovascular, AAA, TAA

1. Introduction

The aortic aneurysm is defined as a pathological condition characterized by permanent dilation of the aortic wall that most often occurs in the infra-renal region and the aortic arch. It generally presents asymptomatically, but progressive dilation can lead to the aorta rupture until the patient's death of the patient [1].

Based on autopsy studies, it is estimated that about 1–2% of the population has an aortic aneurysm, increasing to 10% in the older population [2]. In the United States, an aortic aneurysm rupture is in thirteenth place due to cause of death [2]. Abdominal aortic aneurysms (AAA) are the most common type, and most of them are atherosclerotic. The ascending tract aneurysms (ATAA) instead of the present as the most common etiology medial degeneration, a process normal in aging, but which accelerates pathologically if the person has other disorders, such as hypertension, bicuspid aortic valve, or genetic alterations [2].

2. Etiology

The etiology of aneurysm formation is not yet exact connoted. Aneurysmal disease main problem is the wear of the aortic wall, which progressively increases its dilation and the risk of rupture [3].

Biochemical studies have shown that there is a decrease in elastin in this pathology as opposed to a more significant increase in the share of collagen, increasing the ratio of collagen to elastin in the aneurysmal wall [4, 5].

Animal tests have highlighted that the aortic wall weakening is also due to the intervention of matrix metalloproteases, which act on the degradation of elastin and the destruction of smooth muscle cells [4].

Infections are an uncommon cause of aneurysmal pathology, with cases ranging from 0.65% to 1.3% of cases. Most are attributable to staphylococci, but streptococci, salmonella, and syphilis can also occur [6, 7].

Fungal infections are sporadic, but there are some documented cases [6].

Among the genetic disorders predisposing to this type of disease, we have Ehlers-Danlos, a hereditary connective tissue disorder, specifically type IV, which induces an autosomal dominant collagen type reduction III [8].

Another autosomal dominant genetic pathology of connective tissue is Marfan syndrome. People with this pathology present a mutation of the fibrillin gene, predisposing them to aortic aneurysms, dissection, mitral insufficiency, deformities of the chest wall, joint laxity, and increased arm and leg length [9].

Another one is the Loeys-Dietz syndrome, an autosomal dominant pathology characterized by arterial tortuosity and aneurysms, hypertelorism, and bifid uvula or cleft palate. To be suspected in cases of aortic dissection or aneurysmal rupture in young patients [10].

3. Natural course

Familial thoracic aortic aneurysms (TAA) grow faster, up to 2.1 mm/year. There are also various growth rates of syndromic TAA. In patients with Marfan syndrome, TAA growth rates are on average 0.5–1 mm/year, while TAA in patients with Loeys-Dietz syndrome (LDS) can grow even faster than 10 mm/year, causing death at an average age of 26 years [11–14].

Descending TAA (DTAA) grew more (at 3 mm/year) than ascending TAA (1 mm/year). Marfan syndrome patients with aortic valve disease and aortic dissection who underwent reparative surgery had TAA growth of 0.58 + 0.5 mm/year for the descending aorta. Factors influencing the growth of aortic diameters over time are hypertension, emergency procedures, and aortic dissection [15].

The dissection risk or rupture hazard increases rapidly when the aorta diameter is >60 mm for ATAA and > 70 mm for DTAA. Although dissection can occur in patients with a small aorta, the individual risk is very small [16].

AAA has a very long estimated asymptomatic growth period of approximately 1–6 mm/year. Several risk factors may contribute to its growth and progression such as genetic and environmental factors, among which smoking stands out as a determinant for rapid growth. The growth rate of the aneurysm increases in proportion to its size. Diameter has an exponential effect on the risk of rupture and women have a greater risk of rupture at diameters 10 mm smaller than men [17].

4. Clinic

An accurate anamnesis and objective examination must be performed. Most aneurysms are incidentalomas, occasional findings, highlighting chronicity, and growth rate. It investigates whether you are faced with a smoker if you have experienced weight loss, abdominal pain, fever, or intestinal bleeding over time. It is necessary to study the person from the renal point of view, as a situation of moderate or severe renal failure increases the morbidity and mortality of the subject. The patient's abdomen's objective examination is performed to see if a pulsatile abdominal mass is appreciated. Also, a cardiological objective examination is performed for arrhythmias or valve defects [18].

For this pathology's diagnostic and therapeutic treatment, a division between thoracic aorta aneurysms and abdominal aneurysms is performed. This dichotomy is artificial, as there are thoracoabdominal aneurysms and the possibility of multiple lesions in both areas. The presence of an aortic aneurysm can be associated with aneurysms in other regions. During diagnostic tests, aneurysms of the iliac vessels can also be observed, but those of the popliteal vessels can escape instead. Some studies report that the prevalence of popliteal aneurysms on aortic aneurysm pathology maybe 14% [19].

People with TAA are often asymptomatic, and the diagnosis is often supported by images taken for other reasons or screening. In Marfan syndrome, aortic widening is generally maximum in Valsalva sinuses, responsible for anuloaortic ectasia [20].

Asymptomatic patient is also present in the abdominal aortic aneurysm. The sensitivity of the objective examination is low. People may present with atypical abdominal pain or lumbar pain, but it is not enough to alarm us for this pathology.

Acute abdominal pain with shock is often present in cases of aneurysmal rupture. Ultrasonography is an excellent tool for screening and surveillance, with no proven risks and low costs. It becomes useful during echocardiography to evaluate aortic necessary for the future investigated by other diagnostic tools [21].

The CT scan with intravenous contrast medium (IV contrast) is the diagnostic method for intervention planning. It also allows you to create a virtual angiogram with 3D reconstructions to study the organ ratios. It can also evaluate the coexistence of aneurysms or occlusive pathology at the level of the iliac or femoral artery sectors [22].

MRI with contrast medium, and without it, is the main examination in patients allergic to IV contrast or case of pregnancy of the patient and allows an accurate study of soft tissue, although it does not show calcifications within the aortic wall.

5. Intervention criteria

For the ATAA, the intervention is based on the diameter of the vessel and the patient's medical history, evaluating the risks and benefits of surgical intervention in the election. The surgery should be performed in patients with Marfan syndrome and a maximum diameter greater than or equal to 50 mm [23].

Diameters of 45 mm may be considered eligible for surgery in cases with multiple risk factors such as the family history of aortic dissection, increased diameter > 3 mm/year, severe aortic regurgitation, or desire for pregnancy [24].

Surgery should be considered in patients with a bicuspid aortic valve with a diameter greater than or equal to 55 mm. The limit may drop to 50 mm in patients with multiple risk factors, such as hypertension, aortic coarctation, familiarity, or a 3 mm/year increase in aneurysmal diameter. Without considering etiology, the surgery should be performed in patients with an aortic diameter greater than or equal to 55 mm.

The treatment is also indicated in patients with saccular aneurysms, pseudoaneurysms, symptomatic aneurysms and is also recommended for patients who need valve surgery, considering eligible those who have formations with diameters greater or equal to 45 mm [25, 26].

In aortic arch aneurysms, the surgery is performed for diameters greater than or equal to 55 mm or where the compressive symptomatology is very evident.

The decision must be accompanied by postoperative risk assessment, as replacement surgery is associated with increased mortality and stroke possibilities [27].

In descending aortic aneurysms, the use of stent-graft positioned by endovascular technique prevails. Endovascular surgery should be considered for aneurysms with a diameter greater than or equal to 55 mm. In cases where an open procedure must be performed, the indications are for diameters greater than or equal to 60 mm. Lower limits should be considered in patients with Marfan syndrome [28].

We recommend periodic ultrasound monitoring in AAA until it reaches diameters more significant than 55 mm, if it becomes symptomatic or if it increases its growth rate to values >10 mm/year [29].

6. Treatment

Until the advent of endovascular surgery, open surgery was the only possibility of treatment in cases of descending thoracic aortic aneurysm. Postoperative mortality from open surgery was 10% [30].

Over 40% of patients experience perioperative cardiopulmonary complications. According to some authors, perioperative mortality is about 3%, and the risk of complications like paraplegia increasing values between 0 and 4%. That is true in the open and the endovascular approach, and it may be due to spinal cord ischemia [31].

Since the use of stent-graft for endovascular surgery has been approved, this method has increasingly replaced open techniques. Post-operative mortality has decreased between 1.5% and 7%, with paraplegia risk between 1% and 3% [32, 33].

Open surgery should be considered in young patients with a low risk of perioperative complications.

Successful endovascular surgery depends on proximal implantation, distal to the left subclavian artery, and distal to the thoracic aorta or extending to the abdominal aorta above the celiac tripod. It is generally performed with one or more stent-graft tubes, and the choice of devices depends on the surgeon's anatomical characteristics and experience.

Open surgery remains an essential treatment for patients with altered anatomy, in young patients with few comorbidities, and in genetic collagen disorders. The operation involves replacing the aortic aneurysmal portion with a tube graft, performed by left thoracotomy [31].

During the clamping, perfusion is maintained by right or left cardiac by-pass, allowing for less postoperative morbidity and mortality [34].

With the left by-pass, the oxygenated blood is taken directly from the left pulmonary vein or left atrium and infused by the femoral artery's cannulation. The right by-pass allows greater hemodynamic control but requires higher levels of heparinization and therefore bleeding. The distal clamp is placed just below the proximal anastomosis, maintaining perfusion in almost the entire thoracic aorta as the proximal anastomosis is completed.

When distal aortic perfusion is not used, the repair is achieved with a clamp and seam technique, in which the aorta is clamped and repaired in sequence, with attention to speed to minimize distal ischemia time.

During the open operation, the number and location of the segmental arteries involved in the repair are predictive of the risk of spinal cord ischemia. In a wide range of open procedures, spinal cord ischemia was rare if the segmental arteries involved were < 8 but was 12.5% if >13. Before opening the aneurysm sac, the mental arteries are cut or clamped to avoid back bleeding and subsequent theft from the spinal cord [35].

Abdominal, thoracic aneurysms involve various extensions of the aorta, from the left subclavian artery to the aortic bifurcation, all with some degree of involvement of visceral segmentation. Currently, open surgery remains the therapy of choice in the United States. Successful surgery involves replacing the diseased aorta through a large left thoracoabdominal incision. When the entire visceral segment is involved, the renal and mesenteric arteries are reconstructed through a Carrel patch (typically a single patch for the right renal artery, the superior mesenteric artery, and the celiac trunk with a separate left renal by-pass), or a Coselli graft with a branch to each visceral vessel.

A branched graft is preferred for patients with congenital aortic disease, as these patients are at high risk of patch aneurysms. The need for exposure, dissection, and reconstruction of the visceral segment makes the repair of the thoracoabdominal aorta aneurysm technically complex and highly morbid. Postoperative mortality in high-volume centers has been reported as low as 8%. However, the National Surgical Quality Improvement Program and National In-patient Sample mortality was 10% and 22%, compared to 2% [36–38].

Half of the patients suffer from postoperative pulmonary, cardiac, and renal complications [36, 37].

Techniques have been developed to maintain distal perfusion and minimize renal and visceral ischemia during the reconstruction of the thoracoabdominal aorta aneurysm. In most cases, cardiopulmonary by-pass with femoral arterial cannulation is used to maintain distal perfusion. During the reconstruction of the visceral segment, renal ischemia is mitigated by direct perfusion of the renal arteries with cold crystalline solution or blood from the by-pass circuit. Visceral perfusion is also maintained with blood from the by-pass circuit. Besides, mild systemic hypothermia is often used to minimize the impact of ischemia [39].

There are no commercially available devices approved for total endovascular TAA repair in the United States. However, a hybrid type II TAA repair with thoracic aortic aneurysm repair (TEVAR) has been described, followed by open replacement of the remaining visceral segment and abdominal aorta involved. That can be performed either as a single-stage repair or as a 2-stage repair. While postoperative mortality is similar, there is evidence that a staged approach, either when performing a hybrid or open repair, is associated with a lower risk of spinal cord ischemia (SCI) [40, 41].

Aortic arch aneurysms are usually treated in conjunction with the treatment of an ascending or descending aneurysm. The arch is best exposed through a median sternotomy and most often is replaced with a branched graft with an individual branch for each vessel of the arch. Arch replacement is associated with significant early morbidity and mortality and involves substantial risk of neurological complications, both from cerebral ischemia and embolization. In most cases, arch repositioning is performed in hypothermic circulatory arrest. The cerebral blood flow can be maintained with selective cerebral perfusion prior to the degree of cerebral perfusion.

In the endovascular era, 2 techniques for hybrid aortic arch repair using a combination of open and TEVAR surgery have been developed. Eradication of the supraoptic arch involves by-passing all 3 branches of the arch from the ascending aorta, followed by the TEVAR, including the arch. The proximal holding area is in the non-aneurysmal ascending aorta or proximal arch. The alternative approach is the endovascular modification of the elephant truck technique, used for patients with ascending and descending aneurysms. With this technique, the aortic arch is replaced with a branched graft that includes an extension of the distal tube graft. This is extended distally into the descending thoracic aorta beyond the distal anastomosis. The pathogenesis of the ascending aorta aneurysm is different from that of descending aneurysms and abdominal aorta in many cases. It frequently occurs in patients with Marfan syndrome and other disorders of familial connective tissue or bicuspid aortic valves [42].

In addition, isolated ascending aortic aneurysms are rare, as most occur in conjunction with aortic root aneurysms and arch aneurysms. Therefore, ATAA repair is often performed in conjunction with additional procedures [43].

For aneurysms involving root aneurysms, surgery can be achieved by aortic root and/or ascending tract replacement and aortic valve replacement or reimplantation or composite aortic valve, root, and ascending aorta replacement with coronary artery reimplantation (Bentall procedure).

Recently, endovascular techniques have been introduced in the ascending aorta. The Zenith Ascend TAA Endovascular Graft (Cook Medical, Bloomington, IN) is a device dedicated to the ascending aorta that has been used for type A and ATAA dissection. However, its use remains experimental and is not approved by the Food and Drug Administration for commercial use in the United States [44].

Before the 1990s, open surgery was the only treatment option for abdominal aortic aneurysms and, while continuing to provide more remarkable survival than observation, was characterized by high morbidity and postoperative mortality [45].

However, the paradigm of intervention on AAA changed forever after the introduction of endovascular repair of AAA (EVAR), first described by Parodi et al. [46].

Since then, the use of endovascular techniques in treating aortic aneurysms has expanded considerably, and EVAR is now the primary treatment for AAA. Before the endovascular era, surgical mortality after AAA repair was ≈5%. After EVAR adoption, overall operating mortality from AAA repair dropped to 2.4% in 2008 [47].

The rapid adoption of EVAR has provided a AAA treatment option for many patients who are not candidates for open surgery. Instead, they remain patients with anatomical constraints that preclude the Use of EVAR. Young and otherwise, healthy patients may benefit from open surgery due to its longer duration. Also, patients with anatomical features that make it more likely to require revision, such as a highly angled neck, may benefit from an open approach. Finally, patients with connective tissue disorders should be treated with an open approach if possible, since long-term endovascular complications are inevitable in this population secondary to their disease progression. In addition to patients with substantial medical comorbidity, EVAR is preferred in patients for whom an open intervention would pose additional technical challenges, such as patients with a hostile abdomen. For patients who are eligible for both EVAR and Open, a shared decision-making process based on an in-depth discussion of each approach's risks and benefits is essential.

EVAR excludes an aneurysm from the bloodstream through the placement of a bifurcated stent, most introduced through the femoral arteries. The bag's exclusion depends on adequate proximal and distal sealing between the graft tissue and the vessel wall. For AAA under renal, the abdominal endovascular aortic aneurysm operation is performed with proximal fixation in the neck under renal and distal fixation in the common iliac arteries. The graft choice depends on anatomical criteria, the availability of the device, and the experience/preference of the surgeon. While each graft has been evaluated through prospective trials, the direct comparison between graft types is limited. In addition to neck length, angle, and diameter, other features that affect proximal hold are calcification of the neck, reverse tapering, and mural thrombus.

Some devices use suprarenal fixation to improve proximal tightness, where an uncovered stent extends over the renal arteries. Observational studies have shown that suprarenal fixation is associated with a slightly higher risk of postoperative renal complications [48, 49]. When selecting a device that uses fixation above the renal arteries, this difference should be weighed against the potential improvement in proximal fixation.

Sub-renal devices are designed to fixate distally in the common iliac artery (CIA). However, aneurysmal CIAs presents a technical challenge as they prevent proper distal implantation. Surgeons have overcome this obstacle with 2 techniques: internal iliac artery embolization (IIA) and branched iliac devices.

Open AAA repair consists of replacing the aneurysmal segment with a synthetic graft. In most cases, a tubular graft from the renal neck to the bifurcation is enough. However, if the bifurcation or proximal CIA is diseased, a bifurcated graft can be used. The successful repair depends on the exposure of the abdominal aorta and proximal and distal vascular control.

For surgery, the abdominal aorta is exposed through a transperitoneal or retroperitoneal approach.

A transperitoneal approach is performed with the patient in a supine position through a midline laparotomy. It provides rapid access to the distal abdominal aorta and bifurcation. The aneurysm's neck is exposed by packing the intestine into the right abdomen and dividing the Treitz ligament. A retroperitoneal approach is performed with the patient in the right lateral decubitus position through an incision on the left side that extends inferiorly parallel to the right abdomen. The peritoneal and retroperitoneal contents are moved anteromedially, exposing the entire abdominal aorta and the left iliac artery. It provides excellent visceral segment exposure; however, exposure of the right CIA bifurcation can be occasionally difficult. The choice of exposure depends on the patient's anatomy and the surgeon's preferences. Patients with hostile neck anatomy or short neck may benefit from a retroperitoneal approach and improved visceral segment exposure. Conversely, patients with right CIA aneurysms requiring a bifurcated graft may benefit from a transperitoneal approach.

With the aorta exposed, vascular control is achieved. During AAA repair, an aortic, renal cross-clamping position should be used whenever possible. Suprarenal clamping is associated with higher rates of acute renal injury (AKI) and higher overall complication rates [50].

Hostile neck anatomy may require an adrenal clamp position. In such cases, an attempt should be made to minimize renal ischemia time, and the clamp should be moved distally once the proximal anastomosis is completed. Distal control is achieved with bilateral CIA clamping or balloon occlusion if adequate distal control cannot be achieved through a cross-clamp.

Once access is obtained, the bag is opened, the thrombus is removed, and the aneurysmal segment is replaced with a synthetic graft [51].

7. Complications

Any manipulation of the aortic arch carries the risk of carotid artery embolization and subsequent stroke. This risk is magnified in patients with a very proximal implant area, mural thrombus in the arch, or history of previous stroke [52].

Stroke of the posterior circulation can also occur due to coverage of the left subclavian artery or embolization through the subclavian. Before TEVAR performing a carotid-subclavian by-pass can reduce this risk and benefit from improving the risk of paraplegia [53–55].

Paralysis due to spinal cord ischemia is a very feared risk in TEVAR. Risk factors include extensive coverage of the thoracic aorta, preventive AAA repair, and the left subclavian artery coverage. Visceral ischemia can occur with intentional or unintentional coverage of the origin of the celiac artery. An intact pancreatic-duodenal arch may reduce this risk [56].

The large device diameter required for the TEVAR requires a relatively large sheath of 20 to 26F. It is essential to evaluate patient access through femoral and iliac vessels to preoperative CT to minimize access problems. Calcified, small, tortuous vessels are the most at risk. When an iliac rupture occurs, balloon occlusion can be used for temporary vascular control until the artery can be repaired. Reports suggest that 9.4 to 23.8% of patients require non-standard techniques for safe access [57–59].

Fever and leukocytosis may occur in the immediate postoperative period due to activation of the endothelium reacting to stent placement, to be considered in patients with elevated inflammatory markers and pleural effusions with an otherwise harmful infectious analysis [60–64].

Post-implantation graft migration occurs with an incidence from 1 to 2.8% [65]. Indeed, aortic tortuosity and graft oversizing are associated with migration risk [66].

Patients with traumatic aortic rupture may be particularly at risk of graft failure, possibly due to morphological differences in the unhealthy aorta [67]. Endoleak is relatively rare after TEVAR, with rates reported in the literature ranging from 3.9 to 15% [68].

The risk of death is about 4% in patients with uncomplicated aortic aneurysms. The most common etiology of death is myocardial infarction. For patients with a ruptured aortic aneurysm, mortality can reach 80%. The abdominal wall's retroperitoneal incision is associated with a weakening of the lateral abdominal wall muscles, resulting in swelling of up to 15% of patients. Trans peritoneal incision is associated with a 12–20% risk of ventral hernia formation [69, 70].

The para-anastomotic aneurysm risk is about 0.8% at 5 years, 6.2% at 10 years, and is close to 20–40% at 15 years after open surgery. Several factors influence the risk of postoperative renal failure. These include a longer renal ischemia time, the division of the left renal vein, the bilateral suprarenal aortic clamp position, and the use of additional renal artery procedures. In a juxta-renal aneurysm repair study, postoperative transient renal dysfunction occurred in 37% of patients, with the majority resolving by the end of hospital stay [71].

Colon ischemia can vary significantly in severity. It can be isolated to the mucosa of the colon, or it can be transmural. The incidence of colon ischemia is 1–3% after elective repair and up to 10% after the broken AAA emergency repair. A routine postoperative colonoscopy has been performed in centers where the incidence is even higher: 5–9% after elective repair and 15–60% after rupture. The etiology of colon ischemia may include non-obstructive ischemia due to shock or vasopressin medication, occlusion of the lower mesenteric artery and/or internal iliac arteries and/or atheroembolization. Risk factors associated with colon ischemia development have included the type of repair, rupture, duration of surgery, kidney disease, lung dysfunction, blood loss, femoral anastomosis, and loss of the hypogastric artery [72].

Sexual dysfunction is common in patients with peripheral arterial disease. As shown in the DREAM study, preoperative sexual dysfunction in the group of patients undergoing open surgery and, in the group, undergoing EVAR was 66% and 74%, respectively. The data analyzed after surgery show a greater level of sexual dysfunction in the open group and returned to normal after 1.5 months in the EVAR group and 3 months in the open group [73].

Postoperative sexual dysfunctions' incidence in the two treatments was estimated later, indicating 7.4% in open surgery and 4.7% in EVAR treatment, equalizing sexual function at 1-year follow-up in the two groups according to the ACE analysis [74].

Graft infection complicates about 0.3% of all aortic operations. In endovascular and open aortic aneurysm operations, infection rates are low. Staphylococcus spp. is responsible for most infections followed by gram-negative bacteria. Infection tends to appear on average 3 years after surgery. Treatment includes removal of the graft and infected or necrotic tissue by extra-anatomic bypass or in situ repair [69, 75].

Advantages of extra-anatomic bypass include placement of a prosthetic graft through a noninfected field, excision in one or two settings, and easily accessible axillary and femoral arteries for relatively rapid surgery, but the risk of aortic stump rupture with fatal consequences is 33%. Extra-anatomic graft infection can be observed in up to 20% of patients and graft occlusion with limb loss in 27% of cases [76].

The extra-anatomic by-pass is not a viable option when the infrarenal aorta is insufficient to create an aortic stump. In this situation, an in-situ by-pass should be considered with the use of an antibiotic-impregnated graft, an aorta taken from a corpse, or an autologous venous by-pass. Normally rifampicin is used to impregnate the Dacron graft for antistaphylococcal and partially anti gram-negative action. Advantages of using Dacron include easy availability of materials and the absence of an aortic section. The procedure with neoaortoiliac system uses homologous grafts of femoropopliteal vein, which do not need anticoagulation therapy, to replace the injured wall and through the in-situ approach it is possible to avoid sectioning the aorta. Problems with this procedure include the need for a preintervention to obtain the vessel and the possibility that it may not meet the predetermined length [77].

An aortoenteric fistula (AEF) is a connection between the third or fourth portion of the duodenum and the aorta. Most aortoenteric fistulas occur after aortic surgery, making primary aortic fistulas an infrequent condition. The incidence of AEF has been reported up to 4% of aortic repairs. AEF causes aortic and graft infection and can cause bleeding. Symptomatology includes abdominal pain, fever, melena or hematemesis, and weight loss. Treatment includes control of excessive blood loss, peripheral organ perfusion and treatment of the infection.

The treatment option in open surgery involved the use of a bypass to allow resection of the infected tract and repair of the gastrointestinal tract injury. EVAR has also been studied in the setting of aortoenteric fistulas. In a revision of EVAR for AEF, persistent/recurrent infection or recurrent bleeding may occur in 44% of patients following the procedure and with a mortality rate of 29% due to septic complications in most cases [78].

Limb ischemia is a complication that can occur in up to 25% of cases of open surgery. It tends to occur more for grafts reaching the femoral arteries and in the female population [79].

The types of treatment are based on removal of the thrombus by endovascular secondary intervention or open. The most frequent complication in EVAR treatment involves endoleaks, which occur in up to 25% of cases in the postoperative period. There are different presentations of endoleaks. Type I represents incomplete adhesion between the aortic wall and the endovascular device, in turn dividing into two subtypes: Ia for the proximal complication and Ib for the distal one. When present, it must be treated as it is associated with a high risk of rupture due to increased pressure within the pouch [80, 81].

It can be treated with an open approach if resolution by endovascular surgery is not possible. The most common type of endoleak is type II, found in 10–20% of patients. The primary cause is a reversal of flow in the inferior mesenteric artery (IMA) or lumbar artery that carries blood within the aneurysmal sac. It undergoes spontaneous reslution in 50–60% of cases within 30 days [82].

Type II endoleaks were not associated with an increased risk of sac rupture, so they should not be treated. However, surgical treatment will be necessary in type II endoleaks if they are associated with increased pressure in the aneurysmal sac or if they do not spontaneously recede. They can be treated by retrograde trans arterial catheterization, direct puncture of the sac, or by laparoscopy.

Patients with type II endoleak had more significant complications (death, rupture, reintervention, or conversion to open surgery) and increased aneurysm sac enlargement. Type II endoleak was determined as a risk factor for the growth of the aneurysm diameter greater than 5 mm, especially if type II endoleak persisted for more than 6 months and was recurrent or associated with a type I and/or III endoleak [83].

A type III endoleak arises from a poor seal between the components or from a separation of the frank components. It is associated with the sacralization of the aneurysm and increased risk of rupture.

It must be treated when found. It can be treated either with a stent replacement for low leakage or with aortoiliac devices and a femoral-femoral by-pass for component separation.

A type IV endoleak refers to diffuse contrast redness seen occasionally immediately after implantation. It reflects the porosity of the graft material and is usually self-limiting and does not require treatment. Endoleak, also called type V endoleak, occurs when an aneurysm sac continues to be pressurized, and there is no exact source of endoleak. Management options include endograft realignment, open conversion with explantation and lumbar/IMA supervision if the culprit is found, or explantation with open surgery.

Aneurysm rupture after EVAR continues to be a significant driver of frequent postoperative follow-up in EVAR patients. The ACE study found a 2% incidence of aneurysm rupture after EVAR. Risk factors for aneurysm rupture included type Ia and III endoleak, graft migration, and graft bending [84].

Intermittent claudication after EVAR is usually related to the coverage of the hypogastric arteries by the stent. The ACE study found a 14% incidence of claudication after EVARs. In most patients, it usually resolves over time; however, in about 15% of patients, this complication persists [74, 85].

Author details

Luciano Izzo[1]*, Daniela Messineo[2], Emiliano Venditti[2], Virgilio Nicolanti[1], Sara Izzo[3] and Paolo Izzo[1]

1 "Sapienza" University of Rome, Department of Surgery "Pietro Valdoni", Policlinico "Umberto I", Rome, Italy

2 Department of Radiological Sciences, Oncology and Pathology, Sapienza University, Rome, Italy

3 Human Neurosciences Department Neurosurgery Division "Sapienza" University, Italy

*Address all correspondence to: luciano.izzo@uniroma1.it

References

[1] Davis FM, Daugherty A, Lu HS. Updates of Recent Aortic Aneurysm Research. *Arterioscler Thromb Vasc Biol*. 2019;39(3):e83-e90. doi:10.1161/ATVBAHA.119.312000

[2] Ladich E, Yahagi K, Romero ME, Virmani R. Vascular diseases: aortitis, aortic aneurysms, and vascular calcification. *Cardiovasc Pathol*. 2016;25(5):432-441. doi:10.1016/j.carpath.2016.07.002

[3] Golledge J, Muller J, Daugherty A, Norman P. Abdominal aortic aneurysm: pathogenesis and implications for management. *Arterioscler Thromb Vasc Biol*. 2006;26(12):2605-2613. doi:10.1161/01.ATV.0000245819.32762.cb

[4] van Vlijmen-van Keulen CJ, Pals G, Rauwerda JA. Familial abdominal aortic aneurysm: a systematic review of a genetic background. *Eur J Vasc Endovasc Surg*. 2002;24(2):105-116. doi:10.1053/ejvs.2002.1692

[5] Wills A, Thompson MM, Crowther M, Sayers RD, Bell PR. Pathogenesis of abdominal aortic aneurysms--cellular and biochemical mechanisms. *Eur J Vasc Endovasc Surg*. 1996;12(4):391-400. doi:10.1016/s1078-5884(96)80002-5

[6] Vallejo N, Picardo NE, Bourke P, et al. The changing management of primary mycotic aortic aneurysms. *J Vasc Surg*. 2011;54(2):334-340. doi:10.1016/j.jvs.2010.12.066

[7] Kyriakides C, Kan Y, Kerle M, Cheshire NJ, Mansfield AO, Wolfe JH. 11-year experience with anatomical and extra-anatomical repair of mycotic aortic aneurysms. *Eur J Vasc Endovasc Surg*. 2004;27(6):585-589. doi:10.1016/j.ejvs.2004.02.024

[8] Watanabe A, Shimada T. Vascular type of Ehlers-Danlos syndrome. *J Nippon Med Sch*. 2008;75(5):254-261. doi:10.1272/jnms.75.254

[9] Milewicz DM, Dietz HC, Miller DC. Treatment of aortic disease in patients with Marfan syndrome. *Circulation*. 2005;111(11):e150-e157. doi:10.1161/01.CIR.0000155243.70456.F4

[10] Loeys BL, Schwarze U, Holm T, et al. Aneurysm syndromes caused by mutations in the TGF-beta receptor. *N Engl J Med*. 2006;355(8):788-798. doi:10.1056/NEJMoa055695

[11] Blockmans D, de Ceuninck L, Vanderschueren S, Knockaert D, Mortelmans L, Bobbaers H. Repetitive 18F-fluorodeoxyglucose positron emission tomography in giant cell arteritis: a prospective study of 35 patients. *Arthritis Rheum*. 2006;55(1):131-137. doi:10.1002/art.21699

[12] Albornoz G, Coady MA, Roberts M, et al. Familial thoracic aortic aneurysms and dissections--incidence, modes of inheritance, and phenotypic patterns. *Ann Thorac Surg*. 2006;82(4):1400-1405. doi:10.1016/j.athoracsur.2006.04.098

[13] Kuzmik GA, Sang AX, Elefteriades JA. Natural history of thoracic aortic aneurysms. *J Vasc Surg*. 2012;56(2):565-571. doi:10.1016/j.jvs.2012.04.053

[14] Detaint D, Michelena HI, Nkomo VT, Vahanian A, Jondeau G, Sarano ME. Aortic dilatation patterns and rates in adults with bicuspid aortic valves: a comparative study with Marfan syndrome and degenerative aortopathy. *Heart*. 2014;100(2):126-134. doi:10.1136/heartjnl-2013-304920

[15] Kari FA, Russe MF, Peter P, et al. Late complications and distal growth rates of Marfan aortas after proximal aortic repair. *Eur J Cardiothorac Surg*.

2013;44(1):163-171. doi:10.1093/ejcts/ezs674

[16] Coady MA, Rizzo JA, Hammond GL, et al. What is the appropriate size criterion for resection of thoracic aortic aneurysms?. *J Thorac Cardiovasc Surg*. 1997;113(3):476-491. doi:10.1016/S0022-5223(97)70360-X

[17] Badger SA, Jones C, McClements J, Lau LL, Young IS, Patterson CC. Surveillance strategies according to the rate of growth of small abdominal aortic aneurysms. *Vasc Med*. 2011;16(6):415-421. doi:10.1177/1358863X11423971

[18] Calero A, Illig KA. Overview of aortic aneurysm management in the endovascular era. *Semin Vasc Surg*. 2016;29(1-2):3-17. doi:10.1053/j.semvascsurg.2016.07.003

[19] Gómez-Moreno S, Sabaté M, Jiménez-Quevedo P, et al. Iatrogenic dissection of the ascending aorta following heart catheterisation: incidence, management and outcome. *EuroIntervention*. 2006;2(2):197-202.

[20] Schaefer BM, Lewin MB, Stout KK, et al. The bicuspid aortic valve: an integrated phenotypic classification of leaflet morphology and aortic root shape. *Heart*. 2008;94(12):1634-1638. doi:10.1136/hrt.2007.132092

[21] Erbel R, Aboyans V, Boileau C, et al. Wytyczne ESC dotyczące rozpoznawania i leczenia chorób aorty w 2014 roku [2014 ESC Guidelines on the diagnosis and treatment of aortic diseases]. *Kardiol Pol*. 2014;72(12):1169-1252. doi:10.5603/KP.2014.0225

[22] Rutherford RB. Management of abdominal aortic aneurysms: which risk factors play a role in decision-making?. *Semin Vasc Surg*. 2008;21(3):124-131. doi:10.1053/j.semvascsurg.2008.05.005

[23] Jondeau G, Detaint D, Tubach F, et al. Aortic event rate in the Marfan population: a cohort study. *Circulation*. 2012;125(2):226-232. doi:10.1161/CIRCULATIONAHA.111.054676

[24] Joint Task Force on the Management of Valvular Heart Disease of the European Society of Cardiology (ESC); European Association for Cardio-Thoracic Surgery (EACTS), Vahanian A, et al. Guidelines on the management of valvular heart disease (version 2012). *Eur Heart J*. 2012;33(19):2451-2496. doi:10.1093/eurheartj/ehs109

[25] Hiratzka LF, Bakris GL, Beckman JA, et al. 2010 ACCF/AHA/AATS/ACR/ASA/SCA/SCAI/SIR/STS/SVM guidelines for the diagnosis and management of patients with Thoracic Aortic Disease: a report of the American College of Cardiology Foundation/American Heart Association Task Force on Practice Guidelines, American Association for Thoracic Surgery, American College of Radiology, American Stroke Association, Society of Cardiovascular Anesthesiologists, Society for Cardiovascular Angiography and Interventions, Society of Interventional Radiology, Society of Thoracic Surgeons, and Society for Vascular Medicine [published correction appears in circulation. 2010 Jul 27;122(4):e410]. *Circulation*. 2010;121(13):e266-e369. doi:10.1161/CIR.0b013e3181d4739e

[26] Riambau V, Böckler D, Brunkwall J, et al. Editor's Choice - Management of Descending Thoracic Aorta Diseases: Clinical Practice Guidelines of the European Society for Vascular Surgery (ESVS). *Eur J Vasc Endovasc Surg*. 2017;53(1):4-52. doi:10.1016/j.ejvs.2016.06.005

[27] Chiesa R, Melissano G, Tshomba Y, et al. Ten years of endovascular aortic arch repair. *J Endovasc Ther*. 2010;17(1):1-11. doi:10.1583/09-2884.1

[28] Patterson B, Holt P, Nienaber C, Cambria R, Fairman R, Thompson M.

Aortic pathology determines midterm outcome after endovascular repair of the thoracic aorta: report from the Medtronic Thoracic Endovascular Registry (MOTHER) database. *Circulation*. 2013;127(1):24-32. doi:10.1161/CIRCULATIONAHA.112.110056

[29] Lederle FA, Wilson SE, Johnson GR, et al. Immediate repair compared with surveillance of small abdominal aortic aneurysms. *N Engl J Med*. 2002;346(19):1437-1444. doi:10.1056/NEJMoa012573

[30] Schermerhorn ML, Giles KA, Hamdan AD, Dalhberg SE, Hagberg R, Pomposelli F. Population-based outcomes of open descending thoracic aortic aneurysm repair. *J Vasc Surg*. 2008;48(4):821-827. doi:10.1016/j.jvs.2008.05.022

[31] Sadek M, Abjigitova D, Pellet Y, Rachakonda A, Panagopoulos G, Plestis K. Operative outcomes after open repair of descending thoracic aortic aneurysms in the era of endovascular surgery. *Ann Thorac Surg*. 2014;97(5):1562-1567. doi:10.1016/j.athoracsur.2014.01.046

[32] Wang GJ, Jackson BM, Foley PJ, et al. National trends in admissions, repair, and mortality for thoracic aortic aneurysm and type B dissection in the National Inpatient Sample. *J Vasc Surg*. 2018;67(6):1649-1658. doi:10.1016/j.jvs.2017.09.050

[33] Davies JE. Endovascular repair of descending thoracic aortic aneurysm: review of literature. *Semin Thorac Cardiovasc Surg*. 2009;21(4):341-346. doi:10.1053/j.semtcvs.2009.12.002

[34] Mohebali J, Carvalho S, Lancaster RT, et al. use of extracorporeal by-pass is associated with improved outcomes in open thoracic and thoracoabdominal aortic aneurysm repair. *J Vasc Surg*. 2018;68(4):941-947. doi:10.1016/j.jvs.2017.12.072

[35] Zoli S, Roder F, Etz CD, et al. Predicting the risk of paraplegia after thoracic and thoracoabdominal aneurysm repair. *Ann Thorac Surg*. 2010;90(4):1237-1245. doi:10.1016/j.athoracsur.2010.04.091

[36] Bensley RP, Curran T, Hurks R, et al. Open repair of intact thoracoabdominal aortic aneurysms in the American College of Surgeons National Surgical Quality Improvement Program. *J Vasc Surg*. 2013;58(4):894-900. doi:10.1016/j.jvs.2013.03.037

[37] Cowan JA Jr, Dimick JB, Henke PK, Huber TS, Stanley JC, Upchurch GR Jr. Surgical treatment of intact thoracoabdominal aortic aneurysms in the United States: hospital and surgeon volume-related outcomes. *J Vasc Surg*. 2003;37(6):1169-1174. doi:10.1016/s0741-5214(03)00085-5

[38] Coselli JS, LeMaire SA, Preventza O, et al. Outcomes of 3309 thoracoabdominal aortic aneurysm repairs. *J Thorac Cardiovasc Surg*. 2016;151(5):1323-1337. doi:10.1016/j.jtcvs.2015.12.050

[39] Waked K, Schepens M. State-of the-art review on the renal and visceral protection during open thoracoabdominal aortic aneurysm repair. *J Vis Surg*. 2018;4:31. Published 2018 Feb 8. doi:10.21037/jovs.2018.01.12

[40] Hawkins RB, Mehaffey JH, Narahari AK, et al. Improved outcomes and value in staged hybrid extent II thoracoabdominal aortic aneurysm repair. *J Vasc Surg*. 2017;66(5):1357-1363. doi:10.1016/j.jvs.2017.03.420

[41] Etz CD, Zoli S, Mueller CS, et al. Staged repair significantly reduces paraplegia rate after extensive thoracoabdominal aortic aneurysm repair. *J Thorac Cardiovasc Surg*.

2010;139(6):1464-1472. doi:10.1016/j.jtcvs.2010.02.037

[42] Isselbacher EM. Thoracic and abdominal aortic aneurysms. *Circulation*. 2005;111(6):816-828. doi:10.1161/01.CIR.0000154569.08857.7A

[43] Beller CJ, Farag M, Wannaku S, et al. Gender-specific differences in outcome of ascending aortic aneurysm surgery. *PLoS One*. 2015;10(4):e0124461. Published 2015 Apr 22. doi:10.1371/journal.pone.0124461

[44] Tsilimparis N, Debus ES, Oderich GS, et al. International experience with endovascular therapy of the ascending aorta with a dedicated endograft. *J Vasc Surg*. 2016;63(6):1476-1482. doi:10.1016/j.jvs.2015.12.027

[45] Szilagyi DE, Smith RF, DeRusso FJ, Elliott JP, Sherrin FW. Contribution of abdominal aortic aneurysmectomy to prolongation of life. *Ann Surg*. 1966;164(4):678-699. doi:10.1097/00000658-196610000-00014

[46] Parodi JC, Palmaz JC, Barone HD. Transfemoral intraluminal graft im- plantation for abdominal aortic aneurysms. *Ann Vasc Surg*. 1991;5:491-499. doi: 10.1007/BF02015271

[47] Schermerhorn ML, Bensley RP, Giles KA, et al. Changes in abdominal aortic aneurysm rupture and short-term mortality, 1995-2008: a retrospective observational study. *Ann Surg*. 2012;256(4):651-658. doi:10.1097/SLA.0b013e31826b4f91

[48] Zettervall SL, Soden PA, Deery SE, et al. Comparison of Renal Complications between Endografts with Suprarenal and Infrarenal Fixation. *Eur J Vasc Endovasc Surg*. 2017;54(1):5-11. doi:10.1016/j.ejvs.2017.02.001

[49] Zettervall SL, Deery SE, Soden PA, et al. Editor's Choice - Renal complications after EVAR with suprarenal versus infrarenal fixation among all users and routine users. *Eur J Vasc Endovasc Surg*. 2017;54(3):287-293. doi:10.1016/j.ejvs.2017.05.012

[50] Chong T, Nguyen L, Owens CD, Conte MS, Belkin M. Suprarenal aortic cross-clamp position: a reappraisal of its effects on outcomes for open abdominal aortic aneurysm repair. *J Vasc Surg*. 2009;49(4):873-880. doi:10.1016/j.jvs.2008.10.057

[51] Swerdlow NJ, Wu WW, Schermerhorn ML. Open and Endovascular Management of Aortic Aneurysms. *Circ Res*. 2019;124(4):647-661. doi:10.1161/CIRCRESAHA.118.313186

[52] Gutsche JT, Cheung AT, McGarvey ML, et al. Risk factors for perioperative stroke after thoracic endovascular aortic repair. *Ann Thorac Surg*. 2007;84(4):1195-1200. doi:10.1016/j.athoracsur.2007.04.128

[53] Feezor RJ, Martin TD, Hess PJ, et al. Risk factors for perioperative stroke during thoracic endovascular aortic repairs (TEVAR). *J Endovasc Ther*. 2007;14(4):568-573. doi:10.1177/152660280701400420

[54] Woo EY, Mcgarvey M, Jackson BM, Bavaria JE, Fairman RM, Pochettino A. Spinal cord ischemia may be reduced via a novel technique of intercostal artery revascularization during open thoracoabdominal aneurysm repair. *J Vasc Surg*. 2007;46(3):421-426. doi:10.1016/j.jvs.2007.04.048

[55] Noor N, Sadat U, Hayes PD, Thompson MM, Boyle JR. Management of the left subclavian artery during endovascular repair of the thoracic aorta. *J Endovasc Ther*. 2008;15(2):168-176. doi:10.1583/08-2406.1

[56] Vaddineni SK, Taylor SM, Patterson MA, Jordan WD Jr. Outcome after celiac artery coverage during endovascular thoracic aortic aneurysm repair: preliminary results. *J Vasc Surg*. 2007;45(3):467-471. doi:10.1016/j.jvs.2006.11.040

[57] Matsumura JS, Cambria RP, Dake MD, et al. International controlled clinical trial of thoracic endovascular aneurysm repair with the Zenith TX2 endovascular graft: 1-year results. *J Vasc Surg*. 2008;47(2):247-257. doi:10.1016/j.jvs.2007.10.032

[58] Najibi S, Terramani TT, Weiss VJ, et al. Endoluminal versus open treatment of descending thoracic aortic aneurysms. *J Vasc Surg*. 2002;36(4):732-737.

[59] Stone DH, Brewster DC, Kwolek CJ, et al. Stent-graft versus open-surgical repair of the thoracic aorta: mid-term results. *J Vasc Surg*. 2006;44(6):1188-1197. doi:10.1016/j.jvs.2006.08.005

[60] Gabriel EA, Locali RF, Romano CC, Duarte AJ, Palma JH, Buffolo E. Analysis of the inflammatory response in endovascular treatment of aortic aneurysms. *Eur J Cardiothorac Surg*. 2007;31(3):406-412. doi:10.1016/j.ejcts.2006.11.053

[61] Ishida M, Kato N, Hirano T, Shimono T, Shimpo H, Takeda K. Thoracic CT findings following endovascular stent-graft treatment for thoracic aortic aneurysm. *J Endovasc Ther*. 2007;14(3):333-341. doi:10.1583/06-1955.1

[62] Eggebrecht H, Mehta RH, Metozounve H, et al. Clinical implications of systemic inflammatory response syndrome following thoracic aortic stent-graft placement. *J Endovasc Ther*. 2008;15(2):135-143. doi:10.1583/07-2284.1

[63] Sakai T, Dake MD, Semba CP, et al. Descending thoracic aortic aneurysm: thoracic CT findings after endovascular stent-graft placement. *Radiology*. 1999;212(1):169-174. doi:10.1148/radiology.212.1.r99jl37169

[64] Schoder M, Cartes-Zumelzu F, Grabenwöger M, et al. Elective endovascular stent-graft repair of atherosclerotic thoracic aortic aneurysms: clinical results and midterm follow-up. *AJR Am J Roentgenol*. 2003;180(3):709-715. doi:10.2214/ajr.180.3.1800709

[65] Makaroun MS, Dillavou ED, Wheatley GH, Cambria RP; Gore TAG Investigators. Five-year results of endovascular treatment with the Gore TAG device compared with open repair of thoracic aortic aneurysms. *J Vasc Surg*. 2008;47(5):912-918. doi:10.1016/j.jvs.2007.12.006

[66] Sternbergh WC 3rd, Money SR, Greenberg RK, Chuter TA; Zenith Investigators. Influence of endograft oversizing on device migration, endoleak, aneurysm shrinkage, and aortic neck dilation: results from the Zenith Multicenter Trial. *J Vasc Surg*. 2004;39(1):20-26. doi:10.1016/j.jvs.2003.09.022

[67] Tadros RO, Lipsitz EC, Chaer RA, Faries PL, Marin ML, Cho JS. A multicenter experience of the management of collapsed thoracic endografts. *J Vasc Surg*. 2011;53(5):1217-1222. doi:10.1016/j.jvs.2010.10.119

[68] Preventza O, Wheatley GH 3rd, Ramaiah VG, et al. Management of endoleaks associated with endovascular treatment of descending thoracic aortic diseases. *J Vasc Surg*. 2008;48(1):69-73. doi:10.1016/j.jvs.2008.02.032

[69] Chaikof EL, Brewster DC, Dalman RL, et al. The care of patients with an abdominal aortic aneurysm: the Society for Vascular Surgery practice guidelines. *J Vasc Surg*.

2009;50(4 Suppl):S2-S49. doi:10.1016/j.jvs.2009.07.002

[70] Gruppo M, Mazzalai F, Lorenzetti R, Piatto G, Toniato A, Ballotta E. Midline abdominal wall incisional hernia after aortic reconstructive surgery: a prospective study. *Surgery*. 2012;151(6):882-888. doi:10.1016/j.surg.2011.12.032

[71] Dubois L, Durant C, Harrington DM, Forbes TL, Derose G, Harris JR. Technical factors are strongest predictors of postoperative renal dysfunction after open transperitoneal juxtarenal abdominal aortic aneurysm repair. *J Vasc Surg*. 2013;57(3):648-654. doi:10.1016/j.jvs.2012.09.043

[72] Becquemin JP, Majewski M, Fermani N, et al. Colon ischemia following abdominal aortic aneurysm repair in the era of endovascular abdominal aortic repair. *J Vasc Surg*. 2008;47(2):258-263. doi:10.1016/j.jvs.2007.10.001

[73] Prinssen M, Buskens E, Nolthenius RP, van Sterkenburg SM, Teijink JA, Blankensteijn JD. Sexual dysfunction after conventional and endovascular AAA repair: results of the DREAM trial. *J Endovasc Ther*. 2004;11(6):613-620. doi:10.1583/04-1280R.1

[74] Becquemin JP, Pillet JC, Lescalie F, et al. A randomized controlled trial of endovascular aneurysm repair versus open surgery for abdominal aortic aneurysms in low- to moderate-risk patients. *J Vasc Surg*. 2011;53(5):1167-1173.e1. doi:10.1016/j.jvs.2010.10.124

[75] Laser A, Baker N, Rectenwald J, Eliason JL, Criado-Pallares E, Upchurch GR Jr. Graft infection after endovascular abdominal aortic aneurysm repair. *J Vasc Surg*. 2011;54(1):58-63. doi:10.1016/j.jvs.2010.11.111

[76] Lew W, Moore W. Antibiotic-impregnated grafts for aortic reconstruction. *Semin Vasc Surg*. 2011;24(4):211-219. doi:10.1053/j.semvascsurg.2011.10.015

[77] Chung J, Clagett GP. Neoaortoiliac System (NAIS) procedure for the treatment of the infected aortic graft. *Semin Vasc Surg*. 2011;24(4):220-226. doi:10.1053/j.semvascsurg.2011.10.012

[78] Setacci C, de Donato G, Setacci F. Endografts for the treatment of aortic infection. *Semin Vasc Surg*. 2011;24(4):242-249. doi:10.1053/j.semvascsurg.2011.10.009

[79] EVAR trial participants. Endovascular aneurysm repair versus open repair in patients with abdominal aortic aneurysm (EVAR trial 1): randomised controlled trial. *Lancet*. 2005;365(9478):2179-2186. doi:10.1016/S0140-6736(05)66627-5

[80] Arko FR 3rd, Murphy EH, Boyes C, et al. Current status of endovascular aneurysm repair: 20 years of learning. *Semin Vasc Surg*. 2012;25(3):131-135. doi:10.1053/j.semvascsurg.2012.08.002

[81] Vallabhaneni SR, Harris PL. Lessons learnt from the EUROSTAR registry on endovascular repair of abdominal aortic aneurysm repair. *Eur J Radiol*. 2001;39(1):34-41. doi:10.1016/s0720-048x(01)00340-0

[82] van Marrewijk C, Buth J, Harris PL, Norgren L, Nevelsteen A, Wyatt MG. Significance of endoleaks after endovascular repair of abdominal aortic aneurysms: The EUROSTAR experience. *J Vasc Surg*. 2002;35(3):461-473. doi:10.1067/mva.2002.118823

[83] El Batti S, Cochennec F, Roudot-Thoraval F, Becquemin JP. Type II endoleaks after endovascular repair of abdominal aortic aneurysm are not always a benign condition. *J Vasc Surg*.

2013;57(5):1291-1297. doi:10.1016/j.jvs.2012.10.118

[84] Harris PL, Vallabhaneni SR, Desgranges P, Becquemin JP, van Marrewijk C, Laheij RJ. Incidence and risk factors of late rupture, conversion, and death after endovascular repair of infrarenal aortic aneurysms: the EUROSTAR experience. European Collaborators on Stent/graft techniques for aortic aneurysm repair. *J Vasc Surg*. 2000;32(4):739-749. doi:10.1067/mva.2000.109990

[85] Caporale A, Cosenza UM, Galati G, et al. Criteri prognostici associati negli aneurismi dell'aorta addominale rotti [Prognostic criteria in ruptured aneurysm of the abdominal aorta]. *G Chir*. 1999;20(10):393-396

Chapter 4

Aortic Aneurysm: Clinical Findings, Diagnostic and Treatment

Akshay Kumar, Purnadeo Persaud, Ana Francesca Leite, Nathaniel Aoyama, Ruan Matos, Dor Mordehay Avishay, Nimisha Shiwalkar, Vinit Garg, Juber Dastagir Shaikh, Roopvir Kaur and Asim Kichloo

Abstract

The aorta is the largest artery in the body and can have aneurysms, which are focal expansions of the vessel wall that can occur anywhere throughout the artery. These can be classified as thoracic, abdominal or thoracoabdominal aneurysms and can be caused by several etiologies, including degenerative, infectious, and genetic causes. Most aortic aneurysms are asymptomatic and are detected incidentally while looking for other primary diseases with a physical exam finding of a pulsatile mass, or with imaging such as ultrasound, computed tomography, x-rays, or magnetic resonance imaging. When symptoms are present, they are often nonspecific and occur due to inflammation, rapid expansion, compression/erosion of the aneurysm into surrounding structures, or rupture. Uncontrolled aortic aneurysms can lead to fatal outcomes, thus making proper management essential. Management can range from medical treatment to surgical repair based on location, size, rate of expansion, and presence of symptoms.

Keywords: Aortic aneurysm, thoracic aneurysm, abdominal aneurysm, diagnosis, treatment, risk factors, hypertension

1. Introduction

Aortic aneurysm is a heart disease that consists of the formation of a bulge in the largest artery in the human body: the aorta. For a better definition, the dilation must be permanent, localized and exceed at least 50% the normal diameter of the aorta. A dilation greater than 50% and that occurs in a diffuse way, that is, involving several arterial segments, differs as arteriomegaly. Likewise, ectasia is different from aneurysm when compared, since the dilation regarding ectasia shows less than 50% increase when compared to the original diameter of the artery [1].

AAAs tend to dilate progressively over time, while TAAs have a slower expansion when compared to AAAs [2, 3]. The expansion of AAAs can vary greatly from one to another, however, the larger the aneurysm, it tends to expand at a

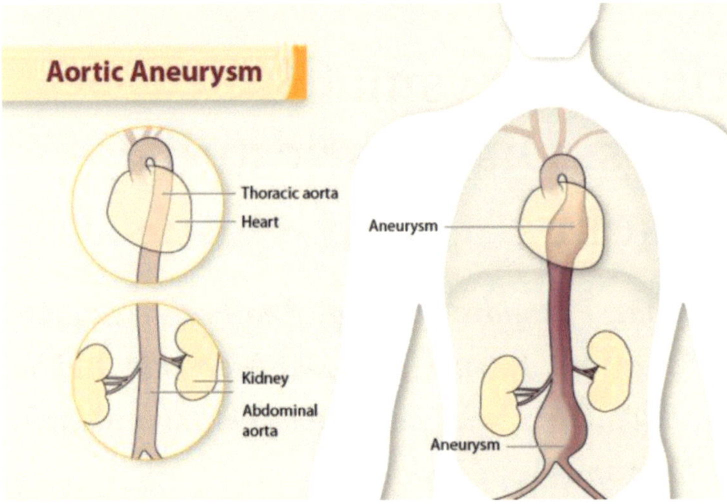

Figure 1.
Different sites of Aortic Aneurysms including Thoracic and Abdominal. (From Centers for Disease Control and Prevention (CDC).

higher rate than smaller aneurysms. In view of the lower growth rate, TAAs tend to be asymptomatic. When TAAs are symptomatic, they are associated with rapid growth, large size and high risk of rupture, which also leads to a higher risk of mortality (**Figure 1**) [4, 5].

1.1 Epidemiology

The epidemiology of aortic aneurysm has several important nuances when it comes to its division for obtaining data. The different types are divided into 8 categories by the Centers of Disease Control and Prevention in the United States of America (CDC), taking into account the location of the aneurysm (thoracic, abdominal, abdominal thoracic or unspecified site) and the presence of aneurysm rupture (ruptured or without mention of rupture).

Table 1 shows that the most lethal type of aortic aneurysm are abdominal aortic aneurysms, followed by aneurysms with an unspecified site, thoracic aneurysms and, finally, thoracoabdominal aneurysms. Also, through the data in the table, we can see that ruptured aneurysms have higher death numbers when compared to the absence of rupture.

171.1 (Thoracic aortic aneurysm, ruptured)	15,254
171.2 (Thoracic aortic aneurysm, without mention of rupture)	12,403
171.3 (Abdominal aortic aneurysm, ruptured)	74,390
171.4 (Abdominal aortic aneurysm, without mention of rupture)	36,233
171.5 (Thoracoabdominal aortic aneurysm, ruptured)	1,784
171.6 (Thoracoabdominal aortic aneurysm, without mention of rupture)	2,937
171.3 (Aortic aneurysm of unspecified site, ruptured)	23,809
171.9 (Aortic aneurysm of unspecified site, without mention of rupture)	13,654

Table 1.
Underlying Cause of Death, 1999–2019 (partial). Centers for Disease Control and Prevention (CDC) [6].

Analysing the epidemiology of AAAs separately, it is possible to extract several pertinent information, such as the predominance of males in the involvement of AAA as a result of screenings studies [7–10]. Abdominal aortic aneurysms have an annual incidence of 0.4% to 0.67% in western populations [11–14].

Deaths due to complications from TAAs, such as rupture and dissection, are usually attributed to other related causes such as acute myocardial infarction for those who are not conducted by post-mortem examinations. This situation is a consequence of TAA being a clinically silent disease [15]. The annual incidence of thoracic aortic aneurysm was estimated in two studies between 5.6 to 10.4 cases for 100,000 patient-years [16, 17].

1.2 Risk factors

There are different risk factors for the two main types of aneurysms. For AAAs, the main factors are atherosclerotic risk factors, advanced age, male sex, Caucasian race, family history, tobacco use, presence of other large vessel aneurysms, food and alcohol consumption. These factors have an influence on both the development of AAA and its expansion and rupture. Another important observation is that tobacco abuse seems to be the most relevant factor to its development. There are some factors that contribute to the reduction of the development of AAA, such as diabetes mellitus and moderate alcohol consumption [18].

For TAAs, there are some studies that show that the factors that predicted TAAs also were the same that predicted aortic atherosclerosis. These factors would be high blood pressure, high serum cholesterol and cigarette smoking [19].

1.3 Different types/causes

There are different types of arterial aneurysms. They are divided based on factors such as location, origin, histological aspects and clinicopathological manifestations [1]. The main study object in this chapter will be aortic aneurysms.

The main division that is used for aortic aneurysm is based on its location. Thus, its division is separated into abdominal, thoracic and thoracoabdominal aortic aneurysms. The first two are the most frequent ones [6].

The field of genetics and how it affects the development of this disease has brought new knowledge about its causes. TAAs may be associated with several syndromes, while AAAs are not [20]. The genetic predisposition of TAA development is well documented. Some of the main genetic influences are Marfan syndrome, Ehlers-Danlos syndrome, syndromic connective tissue disorders, Loeys-Dietz syndrome, as well as other syndromes and nonsyndromic disorders. These are being studied for better knowledge of TAA causes [21].

Apart from genetics, there are some causes that improve the chances of the development of thoracic aortic aneurysms. Some causes worth mentioning are syphilis, aortic arteritis, bicuspid aortic valve, aortic dissection, and trauma [22].

1.4 Pathogenesis

The origins of both of the main types of aortic aneurysm seem to be related to the origins of atherosclerosis in some cases, depending on the area affected [3, 23].

The main alteration TAAs have in the vascular walls are usually cystic medial degeneration. Histologically, there is the loss of smooth muscle cells and elastic fibre degeneration. These processes lead to arterial weakening and, as a result of it, the aortic dilatation occurs resulting in aneurysm formation [22].

In AAA, the extracellular matrix of the aorta is affected by the degradation of elastin and collagen, which are essential for wall integrity. This process weakens the aortic wall and contributes to the formation of the aneurysm [22].

2. Clinical findings

2.1 Thoracic aortic aneurysm (TAA)

2.1.1 Asymptomatic TAA

Aortic aneurysms are often clinically silent if there are no associated complications such as dissection, compression, or rupture. When complications are present, symptoms can mimic other diagnoses. Therefore, it is necessary to suspect a complicated aortic aneurysm in all patients with chest pain [24].

When a thoracic aortic aneurysm is asymptomatic, the diagnosis is usually made incidentally by imaging while searching for another medical condition, such as echocardiography (in aortic murmur), computed tomography (pulmonary nodule or pulmonary embolism), or in screening for the disease in question, in patients who are at high risk for the disease [25].

Regarding biomolecular markers, no specific one has yet been found that identifies the presence of thoracic aortic aneurysm [26–28]. Although some studies have correlated increased levels of D-dimer with the presence of thoracic aneurysm- due to the deposition of a thrombus in the dilatation, newer literature has shown that this product is nonspecific, and can rise in a series of thrombotic events, not only in thoracic aneurysms [29–31]. D-dimer has been used mainly in patients who show symptoms based on its negative predictive value. Moreover, matrix metalloproteinases, cytokines, acute phase reagents, lipoproteins, homocysteine and transforming growth factor beta were also studied, but none of them proved to be a useful predictor in the diagnosis of thoracic aneurysms [28].

Some of the clinical findings related to aortic aneurysm are intracranial aneurysm, inguinal hernia, abnormalities of the branched aortic arch, simple renal cyst and positive family history of aneurysm or aortic dissection. In this sense, patients with these conditions are considered patients with thoracic aortic disease [2].

2.1.2 Symptomatic TAA

The symptoms of thoracic aortic aneurysms are closely linked to rapid expansion, which predisposes dissection or rupture of the aorta. In order to reduce the chance of rupture, if it has not already happened, surgical management is indicated, even if the dimensions of the aneurysm are not extensive.

The most common symptom related to dissection/rupture of a thoracic aneurysm is sudden onset of chest, back and/or severe abdominal pain.

Especially in young patients, it is important that the doctor makes a detailed anamnesis, seeking to correlate the patient's clinical history with Marfan's syndrome, Loeys-Dietz syndrome, Ehlers-Danlos vascular syndrome [15], Turner syndrome, bicuspid aortic valve or other connective tissue disorders associated with thoracic aortic disease. As soon as the TAA expands and compresses the adjacent structures, the pain begins, which may be at the site of the rupture, or in adjacent regions, presenting with irradiated pain.

Depending on the location of the aneurysm, some specific symptoms can be found:

- Heart failure due to aortic regurgitation resulting from dilation of the aortic sinus and annular distortion, in the case of aneurysm in the aortic arch;
- Ischemia or myocardial infarction; due to compression of a coronary artery.
- Continuous murmur that can progress to heart failure, if the aneurysm is located in the sinus of Valsalva and there is a rupture on the right side of the heart;
- Dysphagia by esophageal compression (hoarseness of the left recurrent laryngeal nerve or compression of the left vagus nerve or hemidiaphragmatic paralysis by compression of the phrenic nerve), in the case of large aneurysms that affect the transverse and descending arch, [22];
- Symptoms such as wheezing, coughing, hemoptysis, dyspnea or pneumonitis, if the aneurysm compresses the tracheobronchial tree;
- Thromboembolism or superior vena cava syndrome (swelling of the neck, face or upper extremities), if the aneurysm causes occlusion of the superior vena cava;
- Acute neurological complaints if there is aneurysmal compression of the branches of the vessels of the aortic arch or arterial thromboembolism.

In order to cause symptoms, descending aortic aneurysms need to be much larger than ascending aortic aneurysms. Back pain may occur due to erosion of the aneurysm into the spine, or to visceral or extremity ischemia.

Rupture is the most serious complication, often in the left thorax or pericardium, with severe chest pain and hypotension or shock. If the rupture is in the descending aorta, aortoesophageal fistula and hematemesis may be present.

The association between systemic manifestations (fever, weight loss), increased leukocyte count, and increased D-dimer may indicate a major thoracoabdominal aneurysm [32, 33]. Another two important signs in clinical reasoning are the presence of anaemia, which reveals acute blood loss as the cause of the shock, and high levels of lactic acid due to ischemia.

Patients with thoracic aortic aneurysms that present with symptoms of chest pain are usually submitted to electrocardiography (ECG), which may be compatible with myocardial infarction, signs of myocardial hypertrophy due to long-standing hypertension or valve disease.

The main physical characteristics related to thoracic aortic aneurysms are: Marfan syndrome, Loeys-Dietz syndrome and familial TAA which is associated with livedo reticularis, iris flocculi, congenital mydriasis (ACTA2 mutation) and peripheral vascular malformation [15, 33, 34].

2.2 Abdominal aortic aneurysm (AAA)

2.2.1 Asymptomatic AAA

Most individuals with AAAs have no symptoms, but when they do, pain is the most common, and may or may not be associated with AAA rupture. Like TAA, asymptomatic AAA is discovered incidentally, on imaging studies that were aimed at investigating another cause, or in routine physical examination (especially in patients who complain of coronary, peripheral or cerebrovascular diseases, or during population screening) [35].

About 30 percent of asymptomatic abdominal aortic aneurysms can be suspected by the presence of a pulsatile abdominal mass, which can be palpated on routine physical examination [36]. In addition, asymptomatic AAA is also commonly detected as an incidental finding in imaging studies, and in most cases (2/3) it is not communicated to the patient's family [37].

Another manifestation that should lead to suspicion of AAA is arterial disease due to the presence of another peripheral aneurysm (iliac, femoral, popliteal).

The pulsatile abdominal mass that leads to AAA grows over time, and these dilations are typically asymptomatic, until the catastrophic rupture event [38], where abdominal pain, and even lower limb ischemia due to interrupted blood flow will be felt [39].

2.2.2 Symptomatic AAA

Non-ruptured aneurysms can exceptionally be diagnosed after complications, such as distal embolization and, even more rarely, acute thrombosis. Minor and less specific symptoms include chronic vague abdominal and back pain, which can result from direct pressure or distention of adjacent structures. The recent onset of severe low back pain was considered an indication of impending rupture. Ureterohydronephrosis can also occur, especially if the aneurysm is inflammatory or involves iliac bifurcation [38].

The set of symptoms that lead to the suspected diagnosis of a ruptured abdominal aortic aneurysm: sudden onset pain in the abdominal region or flank (which can radiate to the scrotum), shock and the presence of a pulsatile abdominal mass. Regarding shock, its degree will vary according to the location of the rupture, the size, and the time between the event and the diagnosis.

It is known that most patients affected with AAA are asymptomatic, however, when present, in 50% of symptomatic cases, the classic triad of severe severe pain, pulsatile abdominal mass, and hypotension is present [40]. Limb ischemia or systemic manifestations are also common in infected or inflamed aneurysms [41–43].

The pain varies according to the diameter and position of the aneurysm, whether intact or ruptured, and if ruptured, it may be contained or free. Despite being typically located in the abdomen, the pain can radiate to the groin or thigh [44].

Thrombus embolism or atherosclerotic debris from a ruptured aneurysm can lead to limb ischemia [45, 46], which in addition to the clinical manifestations of interrupted blood flow, can also cause pain. Such clinical manifestations will be apparent if vessels are more affected and arterial occlusion is not well compensated, and may present as sore and blue fingers (blue toe syndrome) or with a cold, pulseless and sore extremity.

Other possible manifestations of AAA are systemic symptoms that reflect the presence of an infected or inflammatory aneurysm or disseminated intravascular coagulation. The main symptoms to be mentioned are fever and malaise. In the case of inflammatory aneurysm, chronic abdominal pain, weight loss and changes in serum markers are suggestive symptoms [47–50].

With abdominal palpation, in some cases it is possible to feel a pulsating abdominal mass and in patients with AAA rupture, some degree of abdominal distension and tenderness will be present [40].

In the case of ruptured AAA, it is possible to find ecchymosis in the patient (Gray-Turner's sign, Cullen's sign, Fox's sign and Bryant's sign) [51]. Moreover, evidence of distal embolization or ischemia on vascular physical examination supports the diagnosis of AAA [52].

3. Diagnosis

Most people with aortic aneurysms are asymptomatic, leading to slow, unnoticed growth of the disease. In this sense, most diagnoses are made by routine exams. These tests are effective in reducing mortality, especially in high-risk populations. Therefore, imaging methods are used, with ultrasound being preferred, as it is not invasive, cheap and generates compelling information, such as the diameter of the vessels [53].

A diagnosis of aortic aneurysm requires an image of this artery to be confirmed. Thus, it is important for imaging tests, both initially and for probable complications, to be taken priority over tests such as ECG, for example [15]. Routine exams, such as chest x-rays on the other hand, often detect aneurysms in asymptomatic patients. Although ultrasound is a priority when a hypothesis of aortic aneurysm is raised, echocardiography, magnetic resonance imaging (MRI) or computed tomography (CT) are great tools for diagnosis, even when done for a condition unrelated to the aneurysm [54].

Expansion of the aneurysm can cause chest and lower back pain, as well as coughing, hoarseness or even difficulty breathing. Abdominal aortic aneurysms, for example, can be checked by physical examination of the abdomen, but the factors for the development of symptoms are not yet well defined, and factors such as obesity complicate this type of examination.

3.1 Screening

Thoracic aortic aneurysms (TAA) are among the top 15 causes of death in the United States. In addition, approximately 1 in 1000 Americans develop TAA per year, 95% of whom are asymptomatic. Data such as these demonstrate the importance of screening for the disease.

It is known that diseases as well as unhealthy behaviors (hypertension or smoking) can damage the heart and blood vessels. In addition, hereditary diseases such as Ehlers-Danlos syndrome and Marfan syndrome can increase the risk of aneurysm. Although the prevalence of abdominal aortic aneurysm (AAA) is high, AAA findings in screening are generally small in size [55]. These findings point to the importance of epidemiological studies and the impact they can have on the outcome of the diagnosis. In this sense, the incidence of AAA, for example, increases sharply in individuals over 60 years of age, as well as a reduction in smoking that can decrease the frequency of this injury [56].

In this sense, it is appropriate to survey the history of habits and diseases, not only for the individual patient, but also for aortic aneurysms in the entire population in question. Factors such as Caucasian race, smoking, men of advanced age and family history are important data to be analyzed for a blunt screening of great importance [3]. Screening, therefore, can change the outcome of the disease, since with clinical and epidemiological criteria, disease morbidity and mortality can be reduced.

The US Preventive Services Task Force conducted a review of the evidence on the effectiveness of single and repeated screening for AAA, as well as its harm and benefits. Ultrasonography, for example, was given as the primary method in primary care for the detection of AAA, due to its sensitivity (from 94–100%) and its specificity (from 98–100%), in addition to not being invasive and of easy execution [57]. In screening, there are some damages that can be observed. Although some data show that women who smoke or have a family history are at higher risk of AAA compared to women in the opposite group, there is insufficient evidence that screening has great benefit [57]; this is an example that even if it looks like a good strategy, it can still generate major complications: the concern about the existence of overdiagnosis and excessive treatment is something of great impact. Overdiagnosis is a major problem in the screening and outcome of the disease-cure relationship of aortic aneurysms, including public health, as it can wrongly consider patients as mild to severe patients, which generates unnecessary or even harmful treatments [58]. In the U.S. Preventive Services Task Force study, it was reported that after the introduction of PSA exam, there was a considerable increase in new cases of prostate cancer. The expected drop in mortality did not occur, and this was justified by the numbers of overdiagnosis, which reached almost 50% of patients diagnosed in the study in that period [59]. For all these reasons, screening is understood as a tool of extreme need, but with the possibility of error and damage in the epidemiological study.

3.2 How to determine the etiology eg infectious vs. degenerative

Whether due to trauma or a pre-existing disease, aortic aneurysms occur due to the weakening of the vessel walls. In this sense, the failure is due to the biomechanics of the aortic wall [60]. Aortic aneurysms have as main factors for development of atherosclerosis, old age and male gender, as well as smoking and family history [61]. For hypertension, there was a 60% finding for patients with TAA [16]; besides that the existence of other aneurysms was also an important factor [62].

One can also mention the characteristics that inflammatory reactions in the vessels can bring. Especially, when considering aortitis, some inflammatory disorders can cause TAA, for example [63]. According to a prospective study by Pacini et al., among 788 patients referred for surgery for TAA, approximately 40% were due to aortitis, proven histologically. In this sense, these factors demonstrate an important causal relationship for the disease.

4. Treatment/management

4.1 Medical management

To this day, for a smaller aneurysm without indication for elective repair, there is no specific medication or other pharmaceutical therapy that is proven to reduce the rate of aneurysm growth or its risk of rupture. Even though Beta-blockers have been advocated to decrease aneurysm deterioration in the past, their effectiveness wasn't proven. Interestingly Doxycycline, an antibiotic with metalloproteinase inhibition action demonstrated decreased expansion rates in animals and humans. However, to this day it is not recommended for this purpose. Nevertheless, addressing future cardiovascular events in patients with aortic aneurysm is recommended. Hence, smoking cessation, blood pressure management, statins, beta-blockers and Angiotensin II receptor blockers are recommended. Alongside, serial noninvasive surveillance of aortic development [64, 65].

4.2 Surgical techniques

Surgical repair is the definitive treatment for aneurysms. It can be classified according to the approach: endovascular or open aortic, or according to the aortic segments: thoracic aorta, abdominal aorta, and aortic arch.

Open aortic repair is aimed to replace the dilated aortic segment with synthetic graft tube. This procedure is done under full anesthesia and it is classified as a high risk procedure. On the other hand endovascular repair aims to exclude the dilated segment from the systemic circulation, by insertion of an endograft. This procedure can be done under local anesthesia and it carries relatively reduced risk in comparison to open repair.

During open surgical repair the aneurysmal sac is replaced with a polyethylene terephthalate graft. The procedure is carried out in a sterile environment under general anesthesia. First, abdominal or thoracic aorta is exposed, then a proximal clamp is placed: below the renal arteries in AAA or distal to the aortic arch in descending TAA, following a distal clamp. Later, the aneurysmal segment is dissected and replaced with a tube graft. Then depending on the aneurysm location visceral arteries are integrated to the tube graft. Finally, abdominal wall or thoracic closure is performed.

In contrast, in endovascular repair first, bilateral or unilateral access via the patient's common femoral artery is established, by a surgical incision or percutaneously. Then, vascular sheaths, through which guidewires, catheters, and the endograft are introduced into the femoral arteries. Then, retrogradely, the "main body" of the endograft is placed over the aneurysmal sac. Finally, the graft is dilated into place with a balloon, and wires, sheaths, and delivery systems are withdrawn. All along the procedure angiograms are used to evaluate graft location, landing zone and patency of visceral/renal arteries.

Alternatively, For aortic segments that involve vital arterial branches (e.g. renal arteries, celiac trunk, carotid artery and subclavian artery) a hybrid technique could be employed. During a hybrid repair, these vital branches are first passed surgically to a proximal or distal healthy aortic or iliac segment, and then an endograft is deployed [66, 67].

4.3 Indication for repair

Elective aortic aneurysm repair is indicated under any one of the following conditions [68, 69]:

- Rupture or dissection
- Acute dissection resulting in malperfusion or other life-altering complications
- Symptomatic states
    - Pain consistent with rupture and unexplained by other causes
    - Compression of adjacent organs
    - Documented enlargement ≥1 cm/year for AAA and descending TAA. Or > 0.5 cm/year for aortic arch aneurysm.
    - Diameter is greater than 5.5 cm for men, > 5 cm for women. Descending TAA with a diameter of >6 cm for men, >5.5 cm for women. While for Ascending TAA, surgical treatment is recommended for lower aortic diameter (5 cm for males).

Importantly, elective surgery, regardless of the modality and aneurysm location over the aorta carries lower mortality and morbidity in comparison to emergent surgery. Emergent surgery is done in life-threatening cases, such as aortic rupture or dissection, and should be avoided by encouraging patients to undergo elective aortic repair [70, 71].

4.4 Complications

Although different approaches of aortic aneurysm repair carry different risks, common complications are hemorrhage, myocardial infarction, renal failure, ileus, incisional hernia, ischemic colitis, embolization, and aneurysm rupture [65, 72]. Nevertheless, it appears that the endovascular repair method carries a lower short-term mortality rate than open repair [72, 73]. However, the biggest disadvantage of endovascular repair is the high risk of complications post-procedure that may need reintervention [74].

An endoleak is a complication that might appear in endovascular aortic repair, in which the graft fails to channel blood back to the systemic circulation. Endoleaks can subdivide into [67, 75]:

- Type I endoleak: an improper sealing between the proximal graft and aorta at the proximal or distal fixation zone.

- Type II endoleak: blood flow from collateral arteries flow to the aneurysmal sac.

- Type III endoleak: separation of stent-graft modular components leading to blood flow to the aneurysm sac.

- Type IV endoleak: blood flow through the pores of the stent-graft.

- Type V endoleak: blood flow into the aneurysmal sac from an unknown source.

Endovascular repair might also lead to access site complications such, perforation, hematoma, and fistula from vascular damage [72, 76].

Technical complications from the graft itself may also occur, with problems ranging from graft migration or kinking in the vessel, to graft infection. The incidence of endograft infection is less than 1 percent, with a mortality rate up to 50 percent [77].

Some studies have shown that ischemic complications are more common in endovascular compared to open repair of aortic aneurysms [78]. Causes of ischemia include occlusion due to endograft positioning, arterial thrombosis, embolism, or arterial dissection and can affect the distal limbs and body organs (intestines, kidneys, etc.).

Spinal ischemia is a rare complication in AAA endovascular repair, and is found in 0.21 percent of patients, but has an incidence of up to 12 percent in TAA repair [79]. This complication can manifest with findings such as paraplegia, pain or paralysis, typically developing within 12 hours after repair [80].

Although this complication is commonly seen in TAA, its mechanism continues to be ill-defined. In one study, perioperative hypotension (MAP <70 mmHg) was found to be a strong predictor of spinal cord ischemia in patients undergoing endovascular TAA repair [81]. Other contributing factors include long procedural duration, previous open infrarenal aortic repair, extent of aortic coverage by the device, endovascular leakage, or thrombosis of collateral blood flow. For spinal cord ischemia, spinal drainage is the most appropriate management, and is also used to reduce the risk of this ischemia [82].

5. Conclusion

Aortic aneurysms have a wide range of possible presentations and etiologies. Uncontrolled aortic aneurysms can lead to fatal outcomes. Therefore prevention, recommended screening, early diagnosis, regular monitoring, and prompt management are imperative to decrease mortality and complications.

Author details

Akshay Kumar[1*], Purnadeo Persaud[2], Ana Francesca Leite[3], Nathaniel Aoyama[3], Ruan Matos[3], Dor Mordehay Avishay[4], Nimisha Shiwalkar[5], Vinit Garg[6], Juber Dastagir Shaikh[7], Roopvir Kaur[8] and Asim Kichloo[9]

1 Department of Cardiothoracic Surgery, University of Pittsburgh, Pittsburgh, PA, USA

2 Kansas City University, Kansas City, USA

3 University of State of Minas Gerais, Passos, Brazil

4 Department of Medicine, University of Milan, Milano, Italy

5 Department of Anaesthesiology, University of Texas Health Centre, Houston, TX, USA

6 Department of Anaesthesiology, Medanta Hospital, Gurugram, India

7 Department of Neurology, Mahatma Gandhi Hospital, Navi Mumbai, India

8 Department of Anesthesiology, Government Medical College, Amritsar, India

9 Department of Internal Medicine, Central Michigan University, Mt Pleasant, MI, USA

*Address all correspondence to: drakshay82@gmail.com

References

[1] JOHNSTON, K. Wayne et al. Suggested standards for reporting on arterial aneurysms. **Journal of vascular surgery**, v. 13, n. 3, p. 452-458, 1991.

[2] Black J, Burke C. Epidemiology, risk factors, pathogenesis, and natural history of thoracic aortic aneurysm and dissection. UpToDate. 2020

[3] Chung J. Epidemiology, risk factors, pathogenesis, and natural history of abdominal aortic aneurysm. UpToDate. 2021

[4] Chaikof EL, Dalman RL, Eskandari MK, et al. The Society for Vascular Surgery practice guidelines on the care of patients with an abdominal aortic aneurysm. J Vasc Surg 2018; 67:2.

[5] Moll FL, Powell JT, Fraedrich G, et al. Management of abdominal aortic aneurysms clinical practice guidelines of the European society for vascular surgery. Eur J Vasc Endovasc Surg 2011; 41 Suppl 1:S1.

[6] Centers for Disease Control and Prevention (CDC). **Aortic Aneurysm.** September 2020. Available at: https://www.cdc.gov/heartdisease/aortic_aneurysm.htm#:~:text=An%20aortic%20aneurysm%20is%20a,to%20leak%20in%20between%20them.

[7] Ashton HA, Buxton MJ, Day NE, et al. The Multicentre Aneurysm Screening Study (MASS) into the effect of abdominal aortic aneurysm screening on mortality in men: a randomised controlled trial. Lancet 2002; 360:1531.

[8] Norman PE, Jamrozik K, Lawrence-Brown MM, et al. Population based randomised controlled trial on impact of screening on mortality from abdominal aortic aneurysm. BMJ 2004; 329:1259.

[9] Lindholt JS, Juul S, Fasting H, Henneberg EW. Screening for abdominal aortic aneurysms: single centre randomised controlled trial. BMJ 2005; 330:750.

[10] Ashton HA, Gao L, Kim LG, et al. Fifteen-year follow-up of a randomized clinical trial of ultrasonographic screening for abdominal aortic aneurysms. Br J Surg 2007; 94:696.

[11] Forsdahl SH, Singh K, Solberg S, Jacobsen BK. Risk factors for abdominal aortic aneurysms: a 7-year prospective study: the Tromsø Study, 1994-2001. Circulation 2009; 119:2202.

[12] Vardulaki KA, Prevost TC, Walker NM, et al. Incidence among men of asymptomatic abdominal aortic aneurysms: estimates from 500 screen detected cases. J Med Screen 1999; 6:50.

[13] Lederle FA, Johnson GR, Wilson SE, et al. Yield of repeated screening for abdominal aortic aneurysm after a 4-year interval. Aneurysm Detection and Management Veterans Affairs Cooperative Study Investigators. Arch Intern Med 2000; 160:1117.

[14] Wilmink AB, Hubbard CS, Day NE, Quick CR. The incidence of small abdominal aortic aneurysms and the change in normal infrarenal aortic diameter: implications for screening. Eur J Vasc Endovasc Surg 2001; 21:165.

[15] Hiratzka LF, Bakris GL, Beckman JA, et al. 2010 ACCF/AHA/AATS/ACR/ASA/SCA/SCAI/SIR/STS/SVM Guidelines for the diagnosis and management of patients with thoracic aortic disease. A Report of the American College of Cardiology Foundation/American Heart Association Task Force on Practice Guidelines, American Association for Thoracic Surgery, American College of Radiology, American Stroke Association, Society of Cardiovascular Anesthesiologists, Society for Cardiovascular Angiography

and Interventions, Society of Interventional Radiology, Society of Thoracic Surgeons,and Society for Vascular Medicine. J Am Coll Cardiol 2010; 55:e27.

[16] Bickerstaff LK, Pairolero PC, Hollier LH, et al. Thoracic aortic aneurysms: a population based study. Surgery 1982; 92:1103.

[17] Clouse WD, Hallett JW Jr, Schaff HV, et al. Improved prognosis of thoracic aortic aneurysms: a population-based study. JAMA 1998; 280:1926.

[18] Stackelberg O, Wolk A, Eliasson K, et al. Lifestyle and Risk of Screening-Detected Abdominal Aortic Aneurysm in Men. J Am Heart Assoc 2017; 6.

[19] Reed D, Reed C, Stemmermann G, Hayashi T. Are aortic aneurysms caused by atherosclerosis? Circulation 1992; 85:205.

[20] Pinard A, Jones GT, Milewicz DM. Genetics of Thoracic and Abdominal Aortic Diseases. Circ Res 2019; 124:588.

[21] Coady MA, Davies RR, Roberts M, et al. Familial patterns of thoracic aortic aneurysms. Arch Surg 1999; 134:361.

[22] Isselbacher EM. Thoracic and abdominal aortic aneurysms. Circulation 2005; 111:816.

[23] Elefteriades JA, Farkas EA. Thoracic aortic aneurysm clinically pertinent controversies and uncertainties. J Am Coll Cardiol 2010; 55:841.

[24] Elefteriades JA, Barrett PW, Kopf GS. Litigation in nontraumatic aortic diseases--a tempest in the malpractice maelstrom. Cardiology 2008; 109:263.

[25] Pressler V, McNamara JJ. Aneurysm of the thoracic aorta. Review of 260 cases. J Thorac Cardiovasc Surg 1985; 89:50.

[26] Wang Y, Barbacioru CC, Shiffman D, et al. Gene expression signature in peripheral blood detects thoracic aortic aneurysm. PLoS One 2007; 2:e1050.

[27] Trimarchi S, Sangiorgi G, Sang X, et al. In search of blood tests for thoracic aortic diseases. Ann Thorac Surg 2010; 90:1735.

[28] van Bogerijen GH, Tolenaar JL, Grassi V, et al. Biomarkers in TAA-the Holy Grail. Prog Cardiovasc Dis 2013; 56:109.

[29] Yuan SM, Shi YH, Wang JJ, et al. Elevated plasma D-dimer and hypersensitive C-reactive protein levels may indicate aortic disorders. Rev Bras Cir Cardiovasc 2011; 26:573.

[30] Diehm N, Baumgartner I. D-dimer measurement: a useful prognostic marker in surveillance of patients with abdominal aortic aneurysm? Eur Heart J 2011; 32:258.

[31] Golledge J, Muller R, Clancy P, et al. Evaluation of the diagnostic and prognostic value of plasma D-dimer for abdominal aortic aneurysm. Eur Heart J 2011; 32:354.

[32] Aboulafia DM, Aboulafia ED. Aortic aneurysm-induced disseminated intravascular coagulation. Ann Vasc Surg 1996; 10:396.

[33] Fisher DF Jr, Yawn DH, Crawford ES. Preoperative disseminated intravascular coagulation associated with aortic aneurysms. A prospective study of 76 cases. Arch Surg 1983; 118:1252.

[34] Braverman AC. Aortic involvement in patients with a bicuspid aortic valve. Heart. 2011 Mar;97(6):506-13. doi: 10.1136/hrt.2009.183871. PMID: 21339321.

[35] Wilmink TB, Quick Cr, Hubbard CS, Day NE. The influence of screening on

the incidence of ruptured abdominal aortic aneurysms. **J Vasc. Surg** 1999; 30: 203-08.

[36] Fink HA, Lederle FA, Roth CS, et al. The accuracy of physical examination to detect abdominal aortic aneurysm. Arch Intern Med 2000; 160:833.

[37] Van Walraven, C., Wong, J., Morant, K., Jennings, A., Jetty, P., & Forster, A. J. (2010). Incidence, follow-up, and outcomes of incidental abdominal aortic aneurysms. Journal of Vascular Surgery, 52(2), 282-289.e2. doi:10.1016/j.jvs.2010.03.006

[38] Sakalihasan, N., Limet, R., & Defawe, O. (2005). Abdominal aortic aneurysm. The Lancet, 365(9470), 1577-1589.doi:10.1016/s0140-6736(05)66459-8

[39] Farber, A., Wagner, W. H., Cossman, D. V., Cohen, J. L., Walsh, D. B., Fillinger, M. F., ... Levin, P. M. (2002). Isolated dissection of the abdominal aorta: Clinical presentation and therapeutic options. Journal of Vascular Surgery, 36(2), 205-210. doi:10.1067/mva.2002.125028

[40] Azhar B, Patel SR, Holt PJ, et al. Misdiagnosis of ruptured abdominal aortic aneurysm: systematic review and meta-analysis. J Endovasc Ther 2014; 21:568.

[41] Kiell CS, Ernst CB. Advances in management of abdominal aortic aneurysm. Adv Surg 1993; 26:73.

[42] Tsai YW, Blodgett JB, Wilson GS, et al. Ruptured abdominal aortic aneurysm. Pathognomonic triad. Vasc Surg 1973; 7:232.

[43] Rinckenbach S, Albertini JN, Thaveau F, et al. Prehospital treatment of infrarenal ruptured abdominal aortic aneurysms: a multicentric analysis. Ann Vasc Surg 2010; 24:308

[44] Assar AN, Zarins CK. Ruptured abdominal aortic aneurysm: a surgical emergency with many clinical presentations. Postgrad Med J 2009; 85:268.

[45] Nigro G, Giovannacci L, Engelberger S, et al. The challenge of posttraumatic thrombus embolization from abdominal aortic aneurysm causing acute limb ischemia. J Vasc Surg 2011; 54:840.

[46] Baxter BT, McGee GS, Flinn WR, et al. Distal embolization as a presenting symptom of aortic aneurysms. Am J Surg 1990; 160:197.

[47] Pennell RC, Hollier LH, Lie JT, et al. Inflammatory abdominal aortic aneurysms: a thirty-year review. J Vasc Surg 1985; 2:859.

[48] Rasmussen TE, Hallett JW Jr. Inflammatory aortic aneurysms. A clinical review with new perspectives in pathogenesis. Ann Surg 1997; 225:155.

[49] Cavallaro A, Sapienza P, di Marzo L, et al. [Inflammatory aneurysm of the abdominal aorta. Study of 355 patients with aortic aneurysm]. Recenti Prog Med 2001; 92:269.

[50] Hellmann DB, Grand DJ, Freischlag JA. Inflammatory abdominal aortic aneurysm. JAMA 2007; 297:395.

[51] David M, Pelberg J, Kuntz C. Grey Turner's sign. QJM 2013; 106:481.

[52] Diwan A, Sarkar R, Stanley JC, et al. Incidence of femoral and popliteal artery aneurysms in patients with abdominal aortic aneurysms. J Vasc Surg 2000; 31:863.

[53] Moxon JV, Parr A, Emeto TI, Walker P, Norman PE, Golledge J. Diagnosis and monitoring of abdominal aortic aneurysm: current status and future prospects. *Curr Probl Cardiol*. 2010;35(10):512-548. doi:10.1016/j.cpcardiol.2010.08.004

[54] Fatimi SH, Panni RZ, Ashfaq A. Incidental finding of a giant aortic root aneurysm and its repair. J Pak Med Assoc 2012; 62:617.

[55] Rylski B, Desjardins B, Moser W, et al. Gender-related changes in aortic geometry throughout life. Eur J Cardiothorac Surg 2014; 45:805.

[56] Safi HJ, Winnerkvist A, Miller CC 3rd, et al. Effect of extended cross-clamp time during thoracoabdominal aortic aneurysm repair. Ann Thorac Surg 1998; 66:1204.

[57] Guirguis-Blake JM, Beil TL, Senger CA, Coppola EL. Triagem de cuidados primários para aneurisma de aorta abdominal: revisão sistemática atualizada para a força-tarefa de serviços preventivos dos EUA: Síntese de evidências n° 184 . Rockville, MD: Agency for Healthcare Research and Quality; 2019. Publicação AHRQ 19-05253-EF-1.

[58] Welch, HG; Schwartz, LM; Woloshin S. (2011). Overdiagnosed: Making people sick in the pursuit of health. Boston: Beacon Press.

[59] Fenton JJ, Weyrich MS, Durbin S, et al. Prostate-specific antigen–based screening for prostate cancer: A systematic evidence review for the U.S. Preventive Services Task Force. Agency for Healthcare Research and Quality 2018, Evidence Synthesis No. 154. AHRQ Publication No. 17-05229-EF-1.

[60] Vorp, David A. "Biomechanics of abdominal aortic aneurysm." Journal of biomechanics 40.9 (2007): 1887-1902.

[61] Creager, MA, Halperin, JL, Whittemore, AD. Aneurysmal disease of the aorta and its branches. In: Vascular Medicine, Loscalzo, J, Creager, MA, Dzau, VJ (Ed), Little, Brown, New York, 1996, p. 901

[62] Crawford ES, Cohen ES. Aortic aneurysm: a multifocal disease. Presidential address. Arch Surg 1982; 117:1393

[63] Nuenninghoff DM, Hunder GG, Christianson TJ, et al. Incidence and predictors of large artery complication (aortic aneurysm, aortic dissection, and/or large-artery stenosis) in patients with giant cell arteritis: a population-based study over 50 years. Arthritis Rheum 2003; 48:3522.

[64] Gowda RM, Khan IA. Thoracoabdominal aortic aneurysm: diagnosis and management. Curr Treat Options Cardiovasc Med. 2006;8(2):175-179. doi:10.1007/s11936-006-0010-1.

[65] David D. Yuh Luca A. Vricella John R. Doty. Johns Hopkins Textbook of Cardiothoracic Surgery second edition.

[66] Chiesa R, Civilini E, Melissano G, et al. Management of thoracoabdominal aortic aneurysms. HSR Proc Intensive Care Cardiovasc Anesth. 2009;1(1):45-53.

[67] Xydas S, Mihos CG, Williams RF, LaPietra A, Mawad M, Wittels SH, Santana O. Hybrid repair of aortic arch aneurysms: a comprehensive review. J Thorac Dis. 2017 Jun;9(Suppl 7):S629-S634

[68] Frederick JR, Woo YJ. Thoracoabdominal aortic aneurysm. Ann Cardiothorac Surg. 2012;1(3):277-285. doi:10.3978/j.issn.2225-319X.2012.09.01.

[69] ESC. Guidelines on the diagnosis and treatment of aortic diseases, 2014.

[70] Kawachi Y, Toshima Y, Nakashima A, Arinaga K, Komesu I. Emergency surgery results in life-threatening thoracic aortic disease. Jpn J Thorac Cardiovasc Surg. 2002 Apr;50(4):158-64. doi: 10.1007/BF02913197 Add to Citavi project by DOI. PMID: 11993197

[71] Timmers TK, van Herwaarden JA, de Borst GJ, Moll FL, Leenen LP. Long-term survival and quality of life after open abdominal aortic aneurysm repair. World J Surg. 2013 Dec;37(12):2957-64. doi: 10.1007/s00268-013-2206-3. PMID: 24132818

[72] Patel R, Sweeting MJ, Powell JT, Greenhalgh RM., EVAR trial investigators. Endovascular versus open repair of abdominal aortic aneurysm in 15-years' follow-up of the UK endovascular aneurysm repair trial 1 (EVAR trial 1): a randomised controlled trial. Lancet. 2016 Nov 12;388(10058):2366-2374.

[73] Conway KP, Byrne J, Townsend M, Lane IF. Prognosis of patients turned down for conventional abdominal aortic aneurysm repair in the endovascular and sonographic era: Szilagyi revisited? J Vasc Surg. 2001 Apr;33(4):752-7.

[74] Daye D, Walker TG. Complications of endovascular aneurysm repair of the thoracic and abdominal aorta: evaluation and management. *Cardiovasc Diagn Ther*. 2018;8(Suppl 1):S138-S156. doi:10.21037/cdt.2017.09.17

[75] Kim HO, Yim NY, Kim JK, Kang YJ, Lee BC. Endovascular Aneurysm Repair for Abdominal Aortic Aneurysm: A Comprehensive Review. Korean J Radiol. 2019 Aug;20(8):1247-1265.

[76] Chaikof EL, Dalman RL, Eskandari MK, Jackson BM, Lee WA, Mansour MA, Mastracci TM, Mell M, Murad MH, Nguyen LL, Oderich GS, Patel MS, Schermerhorn ML, Starnes BW. The Society for Vascular Surgery practice guidelines on the care of patients with an abdominal aortic aneurysm. J Vasc Surg. 2018 Jan;67(1):2-77.e2

[77] Setacci C, Chisci E, Setacci F, et al. How To Diagnose and Manage Infected Endografts after Endovascular Aneurysm Repair. *Aorta (Stamford)*. 2014;2(6):255-264. Published 2014 Dec 1. doi:10.12945/j.aorta.2014.14-036

[78] Gupta PK, Ramanan B, Lynch TG, et al. Endovascular repair of abdominal aortic aneurysm does not improve early survival versus open repair in patients younger than 60 years. Eur J Vasc Endovasc Surg. 2012;43(5):506-12. http://dx.doi.org/10.1016/j.ejvs.2012.02.006. PMid:22386386

[79] Berg P, Kaufmann D, van Marrewijk CJ, et al. Spinal cord ischaemia after stent-graft treatment for infra-renal abdominal aortic aneurysms. Analysis of the Eurostar database. *Eur J Vasc Endovasc Surg* 2001; 22: 342-7.

[80] Awad H, Ramadan ME, El Sayed HF, Tolpin DA, Tili E, Collard CD. Spinal cord injury after thoracic endovascular aortic aneurysm repair. Lésion de la moelle épinière après réparation endovasculaire d'un anévrisme de l'aorte thoracique. *Can J Anaesth*. 2017;64(12):1218-1235. doi:10.1007/s12630-017-0974-1

[81] Awad, H., Ramadan, M. E., El Sayed, H. F., Tolpin, D. A., Tili, E., & Collard, C. D. (2017). *Spinal cord injury after thoracic endovascular aortic aneurysm repair. Canadian Journal of Anesthesia/Journal Canadien D'anesthésie, 64(12), 1218-1235.*doi:10.1007/s12630-017-0974-1

[82] Caton MT, Huff JS. Spinal Cord Ischemia. [Updated 2020 Jul 4]. In: StatPearls [Internet]. Treasure Island (FL): StatPearls Publishing; 2021 Jan-. Available from: https://www.ncbi.nlm.nih.gov/books/NBK539870/

Chapter 5

Complications Associated with Aortic Aneurysm Repair

Zachary Chadnick and Kuldeep Singh

Abstract

Aortic aneurysm repair is a common procedure and may be performed in an open or endovascular fashion, It is important to be aware that there exist many potential hazards associated with aortic aneurysm repair. The fact that this entity can be treated in an open or in an endovascular fashion increases the complexity of the problems that may arise. To begin there exists the inherent risks associated with any surgical procedures in the high-risk patient including bleeding, infection, cardiovascular and respiratory issues that may arise. Complications can also occur in the acute or delayed setting and can present several months or even years after repair. Aneurysms may form in the abdominal or thoracic aorta and each segment has its own unique set of issues that may present after repair. Experience and knowledge of associated problems is imperative for early recognition and best outcomes.

Keywords: aortic, aneurysm, repair, Complications, endoleak, migration, rupture, ischemia, thoracic, abdominal

1. Introduction

Aortic aneurysm treatment can be divided into open and endovascular repair, each with their own benefits and disadvantages [1–3]. The technique is chosen based on the patient's age, anatomy, and comorbidities. Numerous graft and graft materials exist as well. Associated complications vary based on the chosen technique [3–5]. In this chapter we will discuss both acute and delayed complications of open and endovascular repair of thoracic aortic aneurysms (TAA) and abdominal aortic aneurysms (AAA). Factors associated with increased complications and poor outcomes are advanced age, more severe disease, need for emergent intervention with a ruptured aneurysm, and presence of associated comorbidities such as cardiovascular disease (CVD), chronic obstructive pulmonary disease (COPD) and diabetes mellitus (DM) [6–8].

Aneurysms of the various portions of the aorta often have their own unique etiology and pathogenesis and therefore may require different interventions and thus have their own unique complications. Various classification systems exist for thoracoabdominal aneurysms but the Crawford classification is most commonly used (**Table 1**) [9]. AAAs are typically classified based on the proximity or involvement of the renal arteries. Anatomic knowledge and knowledge of the classification systems is important when discussing repair or issues associated with the repair.

Type I	Distal to the left subclavian artery and extending to include the origin of the celiac axis and possibly SMA Possible renal involvement, but does not extend below the renal arteries
Type II	May or may not include part if not all of the ascending aorta Contains descending aorta distal to the left subclavian and extends to the infrarenal aorta, possibly to the aortic bifurcation
Type III	Distal half of the descending thoracic aorta (6th intercostal space) into the aortic bifurcation
Type IV	Entire abdominal aorta from the diaphragm to the aortic bifurcation
Type V	Distal half of the descending aorta (6th intercostal space) and extending to the visceral segment but avoiding the renal arteries

Table 1.
Crawford classification of thoracoabdominal aortic aneurysms.

2. Nonspecific complications

There are several complications of aortic aneurysm repair that are non-procedure specific. Given the common comorbidities associated vascular disease many patients, are at risk for cardiovascular events including, stroke, myocardial infarction (MI), and thromboembolic events [6, 7, 10, 11]. Patients with a AAA are considered to have the equivalent of coronary artery disease (CAD) [12]. Many risks can be mitigated in elective repair by undergoing the appropriate preoperative risk stratification and medical optimization. Patients will benefit from evaluation for concomitant CAD, carotid disease, renal function - especially if the renal arteries are involved [13]. Perioperative morbidity is often due cardiovascular, pulmonary, and ischemic events. CAD is the leading cause of both early and late mortality following AAA repair. COPD and renal insufficiency are also associated with increased perioperative morbidly and mortality [14–16].

Endovascular aneurysm repair (EVAR) is associated with overall lower complication rates compared to open surgery. Systemic and non-specific complications include cardiopulmonary, ischemic, and renal issues related to both IV contrast and embolic disease. In endovascular repair the risk of renal disease ranges from 3 to 12% while cardiovascular complications range from 1.8–5.3% [2, 17–19]. In several studies there are similar risk factors for cardiovascular complications in open repair and no significant differences were seen with respect long-term cardiovascular mortality between EVAR and open repair [20].

The incidence of pulmonary complications ranges from 2.9–3.3% with EVAR, and are thought to be higher with open repair. The need for postoperative mechanical ventilation is as low as 3.0% [12, 17], and the procedure can be done without the need for intubation and general anesthesia depending on anatomy. Many patients undergoing open repair can be extubated immediately after the procedure. Rates of pulmonary complications are associated with advanced age and pulmonary comorbidities at baseline [16, 21].

2.1 Prophylaxis

Patient undergoing both endovascular and open AAA repair are considered to be at moderate to high risk for thromboembolic events therefore use of chemical or mechanical deep vein thrombosis (DVT) prophylaxis is recommended. Incidence of DVT occurs in 1–10% [11] and due to comorbidities, most patients undergoing aortic surgery are at increased risk. Pharmacologic prophylaxis can be omitted in patients who have a ruptured aneurysm as the risk of bleeding is outweighed by the risk of developing a DVT. Of note the use of intraoperative heparin should not be confused with appropriate pharmacological DVT prophylaxis. This due to the late administration as it is often only given after vessel clamping, especially in open surgery [11, 14, 22].

Antibiotic prophylaxis is also recommended to decrease rate of graft infection in both open and endovascular surgery. Bowel preparation is not routinely recommended as its associated with poor outcomes secondary to dehydration. Due to the potential high volume of contrast use, nephropathy can be mitigated by several strategies such as minimizing contrast use and pre-hydration [12, 23]. Renal artery stenting can be used especially in the setting of renal artery stenosis with preexisting renal insufficiency if planning to use a device with suprarenal fixation, although utility is not well-established routine use is surgeon and patient specific [23–25]. Ureteral stenting can be considered in patients undergoing open repair with a suspected hostile abdomen although routine use is not recommended [23]. Lastly hypogastric embolization may be needed to prevent a type II endoleaks or to gain adequate seal zone. With the advent of branched devices use of hypogastric coiling is now decreasing and limited to specific circumstances [25, 26].

2.2 Ischemia

Ischemic complications are frequent and, in some studies, occur at a higher rate in endovascular compared to open surgery, this is thought to be driven by endograft limb occlusion [27]. Lower extremity ischemia is the most common complication and may be due to thrombosis, embolism, dissection or obstruction secondary to malposition [2, 27–30]. This occurs in up to 7% of the patients and occurs within months of repair. Occlusion typically manifests as acute limb ischemia but may present as rest pain, intermittent claudication or decreased femoral pulses. Treatment often requires open femoral crossover graft placement as endovascular technique may not be effective [28, 29, 31].

Intestinal ischemia following EVAR can affect both the small and large bowel although colonic ischemia is more common and thought to be due to endograft coverage of the IMA. Rates are similar with respect to open repair ranging from 1 to 3%. Ischemia in the setting of the SMA is rare and thought to be secondary to embolism due to wire manipulation in the suprarenal aorta [30]. A higher rate of colonic ischemia is associated with ruptured aneurysm, long operative duration, presence of a large IMA occluded during repair and preoperative hypogastric artery embolization [30, 32].

Pelvic ischemia can often occur due to hypogastric artery embolization done either for pre-op planning or incidentally. When patients have difficult anatomy or iliac artery aneurysmal disease the artery is prophylactically embolized. Due to the presence of iliac branch devices utility is now limited. However atheroembolic and thromboembolic phenomena can still occur with attempts to preserve hypogastrics. Symptoms include buttock claudication and erectile dysfunction in up to 40% of patients [33].

Renal ischemia can be due to embolism, thrombosis, dissection or impingement of the origin by the endograft. Incidence ranges from 0.7–18% [34–36]. AKI develops at an average frate of 6.7% which is significantly lower than that for open repair. Inadvertent coverage of the renals by the graft is associated with a short neck, salvage can be attempted by shifting the graft inferiorly, stenting the occluded renals and via surgical bypass. It is unclear whether suprarenal fixation is associated with deterioration in renal function [35].

3. The abdominal aorta

The abdominal aorta is the most common site of arterial aneurysm and is defined by an increase in 50% above the normal size. The abdominal aorta is a retroperitoneal structure beginning at the diaphragmatic hiatus extending to the aortic bifurcation at the level of fourth lumbar vertebrae where it branches into the iliac vessels. It lies slightly to the left of the midline to make room for the superior vena cava (SVC). It's branches from cranial to caudal are: the left and right inferior phrenic arteries, left, right and middle suprarenal arteries, the celiac axis, the superior mesenteric artery (SMA), the left and right renal arteries, possible accessory renal arteries, the left and right gonadal arteries, and finally the inferior mesenteric artery (IMA). The middle sacral and paired lumbar arteries are present as well.

EVAR is one of the most important advancements in vascular surgeries recent history. Using minimally invasive endovascular procedures folded graft components are delivered into a vessel lumen via an access vessel and a sheath. The graft is deployed leading to expansion of the endograft, the graft makes contact with the vessel walls sealing and excluding the aneurysm sac from blood flow and pressure. The endovascular technique has a significant reduction in perioperative morbidity and mortality due to avoidance of aortic exposure and cross-clamping [37, 38]. Although with endovascular repair is associated with high technical success and lower associated complications compared to open repair, the dynamicity of the graft leads to increased rate of late complications. These are related to a technical aspect of the endograft placement such as problems with access, stability or integrity of the endograft the majority of the time.

AAAs are described as infrarenal, juxta/pararenal, or suprarenal renal depending on the involvement of the visceral and renal vessels, with origins below, at or above the levels of the renals respectively. They most often occur between the renal and inferior mesenteric arteries with only 5% involving the renal or visceral arteries. Up to 40% involve the iliac arteries. Infrarenal aneurysms with or without iliac involvement ca be treated easily using standard endovascular techniques however visceral involvement will often require more complex endovascular repair with fenestrated, branched or physician modified devices, or open repair [39, 40].

3.1 Endovascular abdominal complications

Anatomic suitability is the primary determining factor for successful long term endovascular repair. Aortic neck diameter, length, and angulation, taper and infrarenal length are all important measurements to determine feasibility of endovascular repair. In addition to these standard measurements, aberrant anatomy such as renal artery anomalies, horseshoe kidney, iliac artery diameter, distance from bifurcation and sac diameter are all parameters that must be taken into account when planning a successful endovascular repair. With continuing advancements in endograft design their utility and range of use continue to grow. Studies have shown that poor compliance with device specific recommendations are associated with high aneurysm enlargement [41].

The overall complication rate for EVAR is approximately 10% but can range up to 30% in some studies [4, 5, 17]. Endograft complications rarely require conversion to open surgery. Whether complications occur during the initial surgery or are delayed they can usually be managed endovascularly if they require any intervention at all. The main reason for reintervention is typically device related complications. The overall incidence of conversion to open surgery is approximately 2% [42]. Higher complication and conversion rates are associated with larger aneurysm diameter [43].

Vascular access is most commonly obtained percutaneously via the bilateral femoral arteries but can be obtained via femoral cutdown. Open access can be more challenging in obese patients or with prior groin surgery but it may be preferred in patients with severe femoral disease [44, 45]. Prior to device deployment anticoagulation is initiated via weight-based dose heparin to prevent thrombosis and embolic complications, this may be reversed at the surgeon's discretion at the end of surgery if it is deemed the patient is high bleeding risk. Although routinely done, routine use is not associated with improved outcomes [11, 22].

The most common technical compilations include injury to the iliac and femoral vessels vascular injury during access, device deployment or closure. Endoleaks are another common complication and occur when there is persistent flow into the aneurysm sac leading to expansion. Some endograft complications are device specific and will not be discussed here [44, 46].

Contrast related complications such as allergy and nephropathy are unique to endovascular repair and occur at a rate from 0.7–2%. Contrast induced nephropathy is thought to be caused by agent induced renal ischemia causing acute tubule necrosis. Moreover, the long-term use of contrast for surveillance has been associated with decreased renal function in some studies [47–50]. This can be mitigated with dilute use, use of CO_2 angiography and use of intravascular ultrasound for surveillance [24, 36, 51].

Graft deployment occurs after the endograft is precisely placed at the target location, Prior to deployment the blood pressure is typically lowered with a mean below 60 to prevent premature deployment and distal migration, this is referred to as the wind-sock effect. Once deployed the graft is planned at the proximal and distal landing zones as well as at the graft junctions. Evaluation for an Endoleak immediately follows using repeat arteriography. Endoleaks of the thoracic aorta occur at a rate of around 3.9%, lower than the associated rates at 15.3% with abdominal aortic repair [1, 52].

3.2 Endoleaks

An endoleak is defined as the presence of persistent blood flow into the aneurysm sac after graft placement and is one of the most common complications associated with endovascular aneurysm repair. Entire chapters and textbooks have been dedicated to the various types of endoleaks and their management so this will only be a brief overview. Endoleaks occur from inadequate fixation or sealing of the graft, breakdown of graft material, component separations, stent fractures and endograft collapse [52]. There are five types of endoleaks overall.

Type I endoleaks occur when there is an incompetent seal at the proximal (IA) or distal (IB) attachment site (**Figure 1**). Rates can be decreased by strict adherence to the on label instructions for use of the device. Type 1 endoleaks must be repaired if identified and are associated with persistence aneurysm growth. These can be repaired with additional ballooning or the placement of additional endograft components.

Type II endoleaks result from flow into the aneurysm sac from one or more patent branch vessel such as a lumbar vessel or the IMA. Preemptive measures such as embolization can be used and are often effective, however routine use is often not justified or recommended. This is because many type II endoleaks do not require treatment and remain asymptomatic with no effect on disease progression. Embolization, glue insertion, and use of branched devices have all been used with variable success.

Type III endoleaks result from the dissociation of the graft components or graft fracture. Certain grafts are associated with higher incidence of type III endoleaks

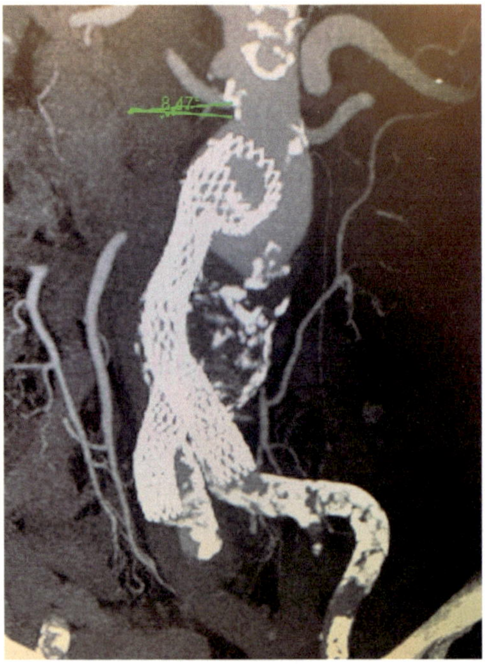

Figure 1.
Type 1 endoleak caused by slipped graft with no fixation.

and thus these can be prevented through judicious device selection. Type IV endoleaks occur due to graft porosity. Like type 1 endoleaks, both type III and IV endoleaks can be repaired with ballooning, additional graft component placement and relining. Both type I and type III endoleaks require urgent intervention while type II and IV endoleaks typically do not require intervention at the time of the initial surgery.

Type V endoleaks are undefined and occur when the aneurysm continues to grow without any demonstrable endoleaks or all imaging modalities. It is referred to as endotension and has no well-defined or established treatment. Routine surveillance using computed tomography (CT) scan, ultrasound (US) and magnetic resonance imaging (MRI) have all been described and various time intervals depending on disease severity. The most common protocols utilize CT angiogram (CTA) at 1, 6, and 12 months with annual follow up thereafter [3, 12, 14].

3.3 Access site and other early complications

Immediate problems are common but unpredictable and are typically correctable at the time of surgery if recognized early. The most common problems are related to insertion of the delivery system in up to 7.7% of cases [53]. Arterial rupture and dissection occurred at 0.7% and 0.9% rate respectively. Problems related to deployment and retrieval each occur at a rate of 0.4%. Accidental coverage of the visceral vessels occurs at a rate of 0.8%, atheroembolism occurs in 0.5% of patients. Lower limb ischemia is due to graft limb kinks and limb occlusion in 0.7 and 0.9% respectively. Lastly the hypogastric artery exclusion is required in 2.7% of patients.

Access site problems during EVAR are among the most common complications at a rate of 9–16% [53–55], these include, hematoma, thrombosis of the access vessel, distal embolization, dissection, pseudoaneurysm and formation of an arteriovenous fistula. Due to the unique pathophysiology and varying severity of these complications they are all managed in their own unique ways. Percutaneous access prevents the need for femoral cut down and thus increases the rate of wound infection. With the advent of new devices and delivery systems there are reduced complication rates compared to the original devices and are now as low as 4.4%.

3.4 Late complications

Although graft thrombosis can occur in the early post-operative period the endograft is a dynamic entity and may respond as such. Late endograft complications occur in up to 30% of cases leading to angulation, kink, migration and thrombosis of the endograft [56, 57]. Larger neck diameter is also associated with adverse events. Migration of the endograft can be identified on abdominal plain films and should be further evaluated with CT [58].

Device migration is one of the most common causes of secondary intervention after EVAR and is due proximal neck dilation either secondary to continued degeneration or oversizing [43, 59]. Another late complication is component separation and is due to the modular design of the endografts. Although the prevalence has decreased with the newer endografts, it can still occur due to inadequate overlap and poor graft integrity. Shrinking of the aneurysm sack can also lead to changes in the forces pulling at the limbs causing movement, decreasing the overlapping length and eventually separation (type III endoleak).

Limb Kinking and occlusion are more common in endovascular repair at a rate of 2.3% vs. 0.2% of open cases. Some studies have shown rates as high as 3.7% and an association with endoleaks, graft thrombosis, migration and need for conversion to open repair. Diagnosis can be made on duplex US, CT or MRI. Symptomatic patients can be treated with additional endovascular approaches and stenting and if the limb remains patient but if occluded open repair and bypass may be required [43].

3.5 Post implantation syndrome

Post implantation syndrome typically occurs in the early post-operative period and is thought to be due to endothelial activation. It occurs between 13 and 60% of patients. This occurs secondarily to the placement of the prosthetic graft and typically presents with fever, leukocytosis and a generalized inflammatory response with elevated mediators such as C-reactive protein, IL-6 and TNF-alpha. With placement of thoracic grafts pleural effusions are common as well, the POMEVAR trial assessed whether preoperative steroids improved outcomes [48]. The trial showed that inflammatory markers were lower in the steroid group, and postoperative narcotics requirements were lower as well. No differences were appreciated in perioperative morbidity however patients fulfilled discharge criteria one full day sooner. No long-term data exists nor does any optimal dosing strategy.

3.6 Conversion

Open AAA have their own associated risks and complications in both the elective and emergent setting. Unplanned conversion from endovascular failure also has its own associated risk factors and is associated with worse outcomes than a planned open procedure. This is thought to be due to the fact that patients may not have been a candidate for open procedure. Due to the known need for conversion to open, when patients are being prepared for endovascular procedures preoperative risk stratification for open surgery is still often recommended [42, 48].

Although many differences exist when comparing open and endovascular surgery the principal distinction results from the need for aortic cross-clamping in open surgery. Depending on the extent of the disease suprarenal and supraceliac control is often needed for at least a short period of time leading to further organ ischemia and hemodynamic shifts. The perioperative morbidity and mortality is increased in conversion from open to endovascular repair in both the elective and emergent setting ranging from 10 to 13% [48–50]. Conversion surgery is associated with higher risk than open surgery [48] however morality rates or comparable and lower in some studies. Late conversion is associated with worse outcomes than early conversion [60].

3.7 Open abdominal complications

Although endovascular approaches gaining popularity for the majority of AAAs, indications for open repair still exist and are mainly due to unfavorable anatomy for EVAR. Open repair is recommended for patients requiring intervention who do not meet the criteria for any endovascular device [19, 20]. Open repair is contraindicated in patients whose procedure risk is outweighed by risk of rupture. Of note, despite the higher perioperative morbidity and mortality associated with open repair, the long-term outcomes are similar when compared to endovascular repair [20].

Factors associated with higher complication rates in open repair are mainly due to medical comorbidities such as CAD, COPD, cerebrovascular disease, and renal dysfunction with serum Cr >2,0, AAA diameter > 6.5 cm, suprarenal cross clamping, advanced age, and female sex. Patients should all receive appropriate preoperative screening and medical optimization including cardiovascular evaluation, Aortic imaging to assess extent of the disease and evaluation for horseshoe kidney or an inflammatory aneurysm which require special considerations for repair [14, 60]. Inflammatory aneurysms are characterized by perianeurysmal fibrosis and contrast enhancing and thickening of the aneurysm wall. An inflammatory component is present in approximately 3% of aneurysms [61–63]. Although these can be repaired endovascularly open repair is often preferred and a retroperitoneal approach is often recommended.

Access to the aorta can be obtained via the transperitoneal or retroperitoneal approach, the former can be further divided into a midline or transverse incision [64]. Although overall perioperative mortality is similar for both approaches [65–67], the retroperitoneal method is associated with lower rates of postoperative complications such as pneumonia, hernias, ileus, reduced blood loss, and shorter ICU length of stay. Retroperitoneal incisions are however associated with increased risk of wound complications including flank hernia and incisional pain. Ultimately incisional approach is based largely on patient factors, and surgeon experience/preference [66, 68].

Anastomotic aneurysms are another complication unique to open repair. They can be true aneurysms related to ongoing degeneration or false/pseudoaneurysms resulting from disruption of the suture line [69]. Suture line disruption can be due to technical error but has a strong association with infection. Both true and false aneurysms can occur proximally or distally and typically require redo surgery for repair. Relining is an alternative if it is feasible and no associated infection exists [70].

3.7.1 Ischemia related to open repair

As with endovascular repair complications include ischemia, and renal dysfunctions. Late complications include incisional hernia, anastomotic aneurysm, graft infection and aortoenteric fistula. Late complications occur in 9.5% of patients [71].

In open surgery extremity ischemia can occur due to clamp injury, wall dissection, thrombosis and distal thromboembolism [19, 21]. Minimizing dissection and clamping heavily diseased regions can minimize extremity ischemia. Pelvic ischemia can lead sexual dysfunction may be due to pelvic nerve dysfunction with autonomic nerve injury resulting in impotence [36].

Renal dysfunction can result from decreased blood flow during mobilization and clamping of the aorta or due to embolism of debris into the renal arteries. Incidence is high with suprarenal repair however infrarenal repair can still reduce renal blood flow and result in renal dysfunction. Renal failure is associated with higher 30-day mortality [25, 37]. The small and large intestine can be both affected in open repair. Acute mesenteric ischemia is rare with an infrarenal AAA. Colonic ischemia is increased with ruptured aneurysm however the incidence of ischemia depends on method used to detect the disease and many patients will not have significant symptoms.

3.8 Compartment syndrome

Abdominal compartment syndrome results in organ dysfunction secondary to increased compartment pressures. This can occur following open or endovascular repair in patients who have a ruptured aneurysm. This is thought to be due to the increased volume resuscitation needed combined with the increased retroperitoneal volume in blood loss. Rates are as high in 10 of patients Following EVAR [72]. Management is with decompressive laparotomy with EVAR and reopening the incision and fascia if open repair was performed. If there was severe limb ischemia, reperfusion of the affected limbs could result in extremity compartment syndrome requiring prompt recognition and intervention with fasciotomy. The myonecrosis associated with compartment syndrome is treated with hydration, cardiac monitoring and supportive care.

3.9 Infection

Infection is rare with some studies showing rates as low as 0.3% in all aneurysm surgeries. Infection rates range from 0.4 to 3% in EVAR and are associated with high mortality rates ranging up to 50% [73–77]. Aneurysm extension in the femoral region can increase the incidence up to 3%. Early presentation is thought to be due to seeding with skin flora or inadequate sterile technique while late presentations are associated with an aortoenteric fistula (AEF). AEFs are caused by erosion of the graft into the small bowel – most commonly the third portion of the duodenum. This is much more common with open repair [73]. Treatment typically requires removal of the infected graft with extraanatomical reconstruction to restore blood flow to the lower extremities. In-situ reconstruction can be also be used [75, 77].

Autogenous conduit such as femoral vein graft can be used and is reserved for use in the presence of gross infection [78, 79]. If the patient does not have an adequate donor vessel antibiotic impregnated grafts, cryopreserved arterial conduits and endovascular grafts have all been used with varying success. Conservative strategies exist with antibiotic therapies if the patient cannot tolerate open surgery. Bloodstream infection and postoperative surgical site infection are associated with aortic graft infection and occur at a mean of 3 years following the procedure [79]. Timely administration of prophylactic antibiotics and adherence to strict sterile technique all decreased the incidence of surgical site infections. PTFE grafts may be associated with increased infection resistance as opposed to polyester grafts.

4. The thoracic aorta

Thoracic aneurysms are much rarer than abdominal aneurysms and can involve one or more segments. Classification is based on the various anatomic structures involved including the root, ascending, arch and descending portions. Approximately 60% of thoracic aneurysms involved the root and ascending portion, 40% involve the descending and 10% involve the arch. Another 10% of aneurysms involve the thoracoabdominal aorta often involving more than one segment.

4.1 Endovascular thoracic aorta

Endovascular repair of the thoracic aorta (TEVAR) is a minimally invasive approach and has fewer complications and associated morbidities than open repair. Mortality rates range from 1.9–3.1% [3, 41, 44, 80], with overall morbidity rates being as low as 9% [42] Despite being its initial use as a treatment for patients who were unable to tolerate an open procedure, it is now the preferred treatment options due to the improved risk profile in most patients with suitable anatomy. Indications for open vs. endovascular approaches are often unclear and many surgical societies place an emphasis on individualized approach taking many factors into account, furthermore many hybrid techniques exist with a combination of open and endovascular approaches [3, 6, 7, 17].

From an anatomical and endovascular standpoint, the thoracic aorta is divided into 4 landing zones (0–4) which determines the need for aortic debranching and endovascular coverage (**Table 2**). Endovascular repair avoids a sternotomy/thoracotomy, and the need to cross clap the aorta. Lack of aortic cross clamping has a lower incidence of end organ ischemia. Endovascular surgery is associated with less respiratory dependency, and has significantly improved post-operative pain, furthermore endovascular surgery has Unless related to a genetically mediated disease, endovascular repair is preferred for most descending aortic aneurysms [81–83]. Like with the abdominal aorta TEVAR can require conversion to open repair in certain situations such as in the case of persistent endoleak and late rupture.

4.1.1 Graft related complications

Various devices exist for thoracic aortic aneurysms. The degree of support varies from device to device and each is thought to have their own benefits and setbacks. Flexibility is associated with increased adaptability to aneurysm configuration overtime while some feel that fully supported endografts are more resistant to kinking ant subsequent thrombosis. Furthermore, increased graft complexity is associated with more complications.

A notable risk with TEVAR is coverage of the left subclavian artery [84]. This is implemented in many patients without sequelae or complications however certain groups of patients may not tolerate coverage. Although routine revascularization

Zone 0	Proximal to the origin of the brachiocephalic artery
Zone 1	Distal to the brachiocephalic but proximal to the left Common carotid
Zone 2	Distal to the left common carotid but proximal to the left subclavian
Zone 3	Less than 2 cm from the left subclavian without coverage
Zone 4	More than 2 cm distal to the left subclavian but within the proximal half of the thoracic aorta

Table 2.
Thoracic aortic landing zones.

is not necessary, patients with a dominant left vertebral system, hypoplastic right vertebral artery, patent left inferior mammary after CABG, functioning left upper extremity dialysis AV-fistula or an incomplete Circle of Willis are at high risk of symptoms including stroke and paraplegia. Any planned coverage in these patients should be preceded by left carotid to subclavian bypass or carotid transposition. Symptoms of subclavian coverage can include development of debilitating arm pain, acute hand ischemia and claudication symptoms. These can be treated with elective revascularization, however may resolve overtime without interventions as collateral circulation develops [85–87].

Depending on the extent of disease the carotid, renal and visceral vessels can all be covered as well. If the renal arteries or superior mesenteric artery are involved the use of a fenestrated or branched graft should be used if possible [40, 41, 53, 88]. If deemed impossible a hybrid procedure can be performed with debranching and reimplantation, or a bypass procedure to restore adequate blood flow. If there is adequate collateral circulation to the covered vessel as occurs with the celiac axis in most patients, no further intervention is required. If not required for circulation and collateral flow exists certain vessels may be prophylactically embolized to prevent a an endoleak [89, 90].

4.1.2 Non-graft related complications

Endovascular procedures require delivery of a large bore sheath into the aorta with separate access for arteriography. This is typically performed via a femoral cut down or in a percutaneous fashion to avoid femoral cutdown. Access site complications associated with TEVAR result from passage of the sheath into the vessel and can result in iliac artery disruption. Rates of disruption are increased if the vessel is small-diameter, tortuous, or excessively calcified. Adjunctive procedures may be performed prior to sheath placement such as angioplasty and stenting to facilitate sheath placement and reduce complications. Other strategies to decrease access site complications are creation of an iliac conduit, directly expose the common iliac or aortic exposure with direct delivery of the graft through the abdominal aorta.

Due to risk of neurologic and vascular complications patients are transferred to a monitored unit postoperatively for routine neurovascular checks assessing for stroke, spinal cord and extremity ischemia. These are rare and in the absence of symptoms, patients are typically stable for discharge after 2–3 days [91–93].

Ischemia secondary to vessel coverage was discussed in detail in the AAA section however ischemia can also occur secondary to embolism during graft placement or from retrograde dissection. Dissection can occur in the immediate perioperative period or be delayed. Rates are as high as 2.5% and are associated with hypertension, vascular disease, presence of an acute dissection and use of bare metal stent [6, 85, 94].

4.2 Ischemic and neurologic complications

The first complication that will be discussed related to thoracic aortic aneurysm repair is paresis and paraplegia. This can occur along any segment and its risk is related to the extent of aortic involvement. It has been estimated to occur at rates between 8% and 30%. The rates of spinal cord ischemia are comparable if not slightly lower with endovascular repair compared to open surgery and range from 3 to 11% [84, 93, 95–97]. Spinal cord ischemia occurs in the acute setting with a mean onset time of 10.6 hours following repair.

There are three major blood supplies to the spinal cord, the vertebral arteries in the neck, the anterior spinal artery and the two posterior spinal arteries that anastomose distally at the conus medularis. The anterior spinal artery supplies the anterior two-thirds. The thoracic spinal cord especially dependent on radicular contributions to the anterior spinal artery, namely the Artery of Adamkiewicz between T9-T12. There are reserves with collateral circulation however as more of the arterial system is disturbed the higher the likelihood of injury. If able to limit the disruption to 8 or fewer segments then the risk of paresis and paraplegia are low. Crawford Type II aneurysms have the highest risk.

Certain spinal precautions can be implemented in both open and endovascular repair to decrease risks. Whether open or endovascular repair is performed, extent of coverage is the highest associated risk factor with paralysis [98, 99]. Hypotension, procedural duration, need for reimplantation and renal insufficiency are all associated risk factors [93, 96, 99]. Spinal ischemia is very rare with EVAR for AAA with an incidence of <0.21% [100] compared to has high as 12% for TEVAR repair. Risk of paraplegia can be mitigated with cerebrospinal fluid drainage using a lumbar drain [99]. Perioperative monitoring using spinal perfusion pressure is also recommended with an intrathecal pressure recommended to be ≤10 mmHg [101, 102]. Reimplantation of patient lower intercostal arteries, namely T8-T12 is also associated with decreased risk of neurologic deficits.

Ischemic complications from TEVAR can occur in the extremities, visceral organs and cerebrovascular system as well. Although less specific to the spinal cord, ischemia to the brain and emboli from plaque/thrombus disruption can lead to stroke and stroke-like symptoms, mesenteric ischemia, and ALI. Overall, 30-day stroke rates were once as high as 20% in patients requiring arch repair but have decreased significantly.

Due to the proximity of the seal zones to the carotid and vertebral artery there is risk of embolic stroke, these are associated with proximal graft deployment, presence of mobile atheroma in the arch and previous stroke. Rates range from 4 to 8% and are comparable with open surgery [103]. Silent embolization is also though to commonly occur however the significance is not well understood at this time.

4.2.1 Visceral ischemia

Celiac axis coverage is controversial and although not typical, can result in visceral ischemia. Collateralization via in the pancreaticoduodenal arcade should allow blood flow via the SMA however this is not always the case. If the graft were to cover the SMA or renal arteries, revascularization would be necessary if a fenestrated or branched device was not used [90, 104].

4.3 Delayed complications

CT Scan is used for surveillance and typically done at 1, 6, and 12 months post operatively with annual surveillance thereafter. Secondary intervention is fairly common [3, 17, 103, 105] and evidence of endoleaks typically require prompt intervention. Type II endoleaks in the setting of stable aneurysm sack size can be observed.

Late outcomes are usually related to the natural history of the disease and related to the graft itself, endoleaks have been discussed but the device can migrate, collapse or infold as well [1, 47]. Migration above 1 cm caudally can occur at a rate of 1–3% over a one-year period. This is increased with grafts that are oversized or associated with tortuous seal zone. In-folding and collapse primarily occur in younger patients and has a higher association with traumatic dissection and is related to severe proximal aortic angulation or oversizing. Symptoms are related to aortic occlusion and require prompt intervention. Overlapping and device separation has been reported as well, however all of these issues typically respond well to endovascular techniques [106, 107]. The need for secondary intervention from various causes ranges from 3.6 to 24% [108–111].

A large case series with 1 year follow up looked at patients treated with endovascular stents for aneurysm, dissection and traumatic injury with fatal complications occurring in 4% of patients resulting from aneurysmal rupture, stent erosion into the esophagus, bleeding and arterial injury [112]. Late stent complications occurred in 38% of patients and presented with malposition, endoleaks, dissection, distal embolization, gut ischemia, and infection. Aortobronchial and aortopulmonary fistulas related to compression as a consequence of endoleaks are rare but potential lethal complications.

4.4 Open thoracic complications

Although endovascular procedures are gaining popularity for many thoracic pathologies, open surgery still remains the standard of care for various situations. Open surgery remains the standard of care for ascending aneurysms >5.5 cm, >4.5 cm with associated genetic anomalies (>4.2 cm with patients with Loeys-Dietz Syndrome), and rapid expansion. Patient selection must also be considered and may be an indication for open repair. As many open thoracic procedures require cardiopulmonary bypass and often use hypothermic circulatory arrest, the associated risks and complications all apply and will not be discussed in detail [3, 92]. In summary patients who do not me the anatomic criteria to place an available endograft and require repair they must undergo an open procedure.

Bleeding requiring intervention occurs in 10% of patients requiring emergent repair and 3% of patients undergoing elective repair. Bleeding can lead to cardiac tamponade, shock, dilutional coagulopathy and have other associated transfusion related complications. It can also present in a delayed fashion with a hemothorax requiring further intervention. Prevention can include correction of all coagulation defects, obtaining strict hemostasis, use of antifibrinolytic and hemostatic agents. Bleeding can occur with TEVAR, EVAR and Open AAA repair however is most severe when associated with open thoracic repair [3, 113, 114].

Ischemic renal and neurologic complications are discussed above however emboli and ischemia can affect the extremities and visceral organs as well. Peripheral nerve injuries can result as a consequence of excessive traction, but often improve with conservative management and do not require any interventions [30, 35]. Distal arch surgery is associated with injury to the recurrent laryngeal nerve resulting in hoarseness and vocal cord paralysis, while injury to the phrenic nerve is associated with diaphragmatic paralysis and respiratory distress/failure [3].

Para-anastomotic pseudoaneurysm is a notable potential late complication of open thoracoabdominal repair, and often occurs in the setting of graft infection. It is often repaired with re-do open repair, however endovascular options exist for certain patients with appropriate anatomy and prohibitive risk to open surgery [69].

4.5 The aortic valve

The involvement of the aortic valve requires special consideration with repair and thus has its own specific set of associated complications. Furthermore, aortic stenosis and insufficiency may present as a late complication of ascending aortic or arch repair. This can also be associated with re-aneurysm formation, dissection and endocarditis of the valve. Furthermore, involvement of the aortic valve and root require coronary artery reimplantation. Valve-sparing aortic replacement is possible and recommended for patients with ascending disease who do not have significant root dilation [115–117].

5. Conclusion

In conclusion many complications exist with respect to aortic aneurysm repair and exist among all types of repair and relate to the comorbidities associated with the disease such as myocardial infarction and stroke, while others related to graft placement and surgery as occurs with visceral ischemia. Endovascular and Open repair and the Abdominal and thoracic aorta each do have their own unique associated risks. Open procedures have high rates of infection and bleeding, while endovascular repair have higher associated risks of contrast related injuries and risk conversion to open surgery. The thoracic aorta has higher associated rates of spinal ischemia and paralysis.

Conflict of interest

The authors declare no conflict of interest.

Author details

Zachary Chadnick and Kuldeep Singh*
Staten Island University Hospital, New York, United States

*Address all correspondence to: ksingh7@northwell.edu

References

[1] Bavaria JE, Appoo JJ, Makaroun MS, Verter J, Yu Z-F, Mitchell RS, et al. Endovascular stent grafting versus open surgical repair of descending thoracic aortic aneurysms in low-risk patients: a multicenter comparative trial. J Thorac Cardiovasc Surg. 2007 Feb;133(2):369-377.

[2] Becquemin J-P, Pillet J-C, Lescalie F, Sapoval M, Goueffic Y, Lermusiaux P, et al. A randomized controlled trial of endovascular aneurysm repair versus open surgery for abdominal aortic aneurysms in low- to moderate-risk patients. J Vasc Surg. 2011 May;53(5):1167-1173.e1.

[3] Hiratzka LF, Bakris GL, Beckman JA, Bersin RM, Carr VF, Casey DE, et al. 2010 ACCF/AHA/AATS/ACR/ASA/SCA/SCAI/SIR/STS/SVM guidelines for the diagnosis and management of patients with Thoracic Aortic Disease: a report of the American College of Cardiology Foundation/American Heart Association Task Force on Practice Guidelines, American Association for Thoracic Surgery, American College of Radiology, American Stroke Association, Society of Cardiovascular Anesthesiologists, Society for Cardiovascular Angiography and Interventions, Society of Interventional Radiology, Society of Thoracic Surgeons, and Society for Vascular Medicine. Circulation. 2010 Apr 6;121(13):e266-369.

[4] Gabrielli L, Baudo A, Molinari A, Domanin M. Early complications in endovascular treatment of abdominal aortic aneurysm. Acta Chir Belg. 2004 Oct;104(5):519-526.

[5] Brown LC, Greenhalgh RM, Powell JT, Thompson SG, EVAR Trial Participants. Use of baseline factors to predict complications and reinterventions after endovascular repair of abdominal aortic aneurysm. Br J Surg. 2010 Aug;97(8):1207-1217.

[6] Coady MA, Rizzo JA, Hammond GL, Kopf GS, Elefteriades JA. Surgical intervention criteria for thoracic aortic aneurysms: a study of growth rates and complications. Ann Thorac Surg. 1999 Jun;67(6):1922-1926; discussion 1953-1958.

[7] Chung J, Corriere MA, Veeraswamy RK, Kasirajan K, Milner R, Dodson TF, et al. Risk factors for late mortality after endovascular repair of the thoracic aorta. J Vasc Surg. 2010 Sep;52(3):549-554; discussion 555.

[8] Feezor RJ, Martin TD, Hess PJ, Klodell CT, Beaver TM, Huber TS, et al. Risk factors for perioperative stroke during thoracic endovascular aortic repairs (TEVAR). J Endovasc Ther. 2007 Aug;14(4):568-573.

[9] Vandy FC, Girotti M, Williams DM, Eliason JL, Dasika NL, Michael Deeb G, et al. Iliofemoral complications associated with thoracic endovascular aortic repair: frequency, risk factors, and early and late outcomes. J Thorac Cardiovasc Surg. 2014 Mar;147(3):960-965.

[10] Crawford ES, Crawford JL, Safi HJ, Coselli JS, Hess KR, Brooks B, et al. Thoracoabdominal aortic aneurysms: preoperative and intraoperative factors determining immediate and long-term results of operations in 605 patients. J Vasc Surg. 1986 Mar;3(3):389-404.

[11] de Maistre E, Terriat B, Lesne-Padieu A-S, Abello N, Bouchot O, Steinmetz EF. High incidence of venous thrombosis after surgery for abdominal aortic aneurysm. J Vasc Surg. 2009 Mar;49(3):596-601.

[12] Hirsch AT, Haskal ZJ, Hertzer NR, Bakal CW, Creager MA, Halperin JL, et al. ACC/AHA 2005 Practice Guidelines for the management of patients with peripheral arterial disease (lower

extremity, renal, mesenteric, and abdominal aortic): a collaborative report from the American Association for Vascular Surgery/Society for Vascular Surgery, Society for Cardiovascular Angiography and Interventions, Society for Vascular Medicine and Biology, Society of Interventional Radiology, and the ACC/AHA Task Force on Practice Guidelines (Writing Committee to Develop Guidelines for the Management of Patients With Peripheral Arterial Disease): endorsed by the American Association of Cardiovascular and Pulmonary Rehabilitation; National Heart, Lung, and Blood Institute; Society for Vascular Nursing; TransAtlantic Inter-Society Consensus; and Vascular Disease Foundation. Circulation. 2006 Mar 21;113(11):e463-654.

[13] Dawson J, Vig S, Choke E, Blundell J, Horne G, Downham C, et al. Medical optimisation can reduce morbidity and mortality associated with elective aortic aneurysm repair. Eur J Vasc Endovasc Surg. 2007 Jan;33(1):100-104.

[14] Chaikof EL, Brewster DC, Dalman RL, Makaroun MS, Illig KA, Sicard GA, et al. The care of patients with an abdominal aortic aneurysm: the Society for Vascular Surgery practice guidelines. J Vasc Surg. 2009 Oct;50 (4 Suppl):S2-49.

[15] Chaikof EL, Blankensteijn JD, Harris PL, White GH, Zarins CK, Bernhard VM, et al. Reporting standards for endovascular aortic aneurysm repair. J Vasc Surg. 2002 May;35(5):1048-1060.

[16] Moll FL, Powell JT, Fraedrich G, Verzini F, Haulon S, Waltham M, et al. Management of abdominal aortic aneurysms clinical practice guidelines of the European society for vascular surgery. Eur J Vasc Endovasc Surg. 2011 Jan;41 Suppl 1:S1-58.

[17] Prinssen M, Verhoeven ELG, Buth J, Cuypers PWM, van Sambeek MRHM, Balm R, et al. A randomized trial comparing conventional and endovascular repair of abdominal aortic aneurysms. N Engl J Med. 2004 Oct 14;351(16):1607-1618.

[18] EVAR trial participants. Endovascular aneurysm repair versus open repair in patients with abdominal aortic aneurysm (EVAR trial 1): randomised controlled trial. Lancet. 2005 Jul 25;365(9478):2179-2186.

[19] Lederle FA, Freischlag JA, Kyriakides TC, Padberg FT, Matsumura JS, Kohler TR, et al. Outcomes following endovascular vs open repair of abdominal aortic aneurysm: a randomized trial. JAMA. 2009 Oct 14;302(14):1535-1542.

[20] Khan S, Lombardi JV, Carpenter JP, Trani J, Alexander JB, Caputo FJ. Open abdominal aortic aneurysm repair is still necessary in an era of advanced endovascular repair. J Vasc Surg. 2016 Aug;64(2):333-337.

[21] Fonseca R, Rockman C, Pitti A, Cayne N, Maldonado TS, Lamparello PJ, et al. Intermediate-term EVAR outcomes in octogenarians. J Vasc Surg. 2010 Sep;52(3):556-560; discussion 560-561.

[22] Gould MK, Garcia DA, Wren SM, Karanicolas PJ, Arcelus JI, Heit JA, et al. Prevention of VTE in nonorthopedic surgical patients: Antithrombotic Therapy and Prevention of Thrombosis, 9th ed: American College of Chest Physicians Evidence-Based Clinical Practice Guidelines. Chest. 2012 Feb;141(2 Suppl):e227S-e277S.

[23] Landry GJ, Lau IH, Liem TK, Mitchell EL, Moneta GL. Adjunctive renal artery revascularization during juxtarenal and suprarenal abdominal aortic aneurysm repairs. Am J Surg. 2010 May;199(5):641-645.

[24] Brown LC, Brown EA, Greenhalgh RM, Powell JT,

Thompson SG, UK EVAR Trial Participants. Renal function and abdominal aortic aneurysm (AAA): the impact of different management strategies on long-term renal function in the UK EndoVascular Aneurysm Repair (EVAR) Trials. Ann Surg. 2010 May;251(5):966-975.

[25] Zettervall SL, Soden PA, Deery SE, Ultee K, Shean KE, Shuja F, et al. Comparison of Renal Complications between Endografts with Suprarenal and Infrarenal Fixation. Eur J Vasc Endovasc Surg. 2017 Jul;54(1):5-11.

[26] Kusaka J, Matsumoto S, Hagiwara S, Koga H, Noguchi T. Use of perioperative ureteral stent in abdominal aortic aneurysm with retroperitoneal fibrosis - A report of two cases. Korean J Anesthesiol. 2012 Jul;63(1):76-79.

[27] Casey K, Al-Khatib WK, Zhou W. Hypogastric artery preservation during aortoiliac aneurysm repair. Ann Vasc Surg. 2011 Jan;25(1):133.e1-8.

[28] Mehta M, Veith FJ, Ohki T, Cynamon J, Goldstein K, Suggs WD, et al. Unilateral and bilateral hypogastric artery interruption during aortoiliac aneurysm repair in 154 patients: a relatively innocuous procedure. J Vasc Surg. 2001 Feb;33(2 Suppl):S27–S32.

[29] Maldonado TS, Rockman CB, Riles E, Douglas D, Adelman MA, Jacobowitz GR, et al. Ischemic complications after endovascular abdominal aortic aneurysm repair. J Vasc Surg. 2004 Oct;40(4):703-709; discussion 709-710.

[30] Faure EM, Becquemin J-P, Cochennec F, ENGAGE collaborators. Predictive factors for limb occlusions after endovascular aneurysm repair. J Vasc Surg. 2015 May;61(5):1138-1145.e2.

[31] Taudorf M, Jensen LP, Vogt KC, Grønvall J, Schroeder TV, Lönn L. Endograft limb occlusion in EVAR: iliac tortuosity quantified by three different indices on the basis of preoperative CTA. Eur J Vasc Endovasc Surg. 2014 Nov;48(5):527-533.

[32] Becquemin J-P, Majewski M, Fermani N, Marzelle J, Desgrandes P, Allaire E, et al. Colon ischemia following abdominal aortic aneurysm repair in the era of endovascular abdominal aortic repair. J Vasc Surg. 2008 Feb;47(2):258-263; discussion 263.

[33] Mantas GK, Antonopoulos CN, Sfyroeras GS, Moulakakis KG, Kakisis JD, Mylonas SN, et al. Factors Predisposing to Endograft Limb Occlusion after Endovascular Aortic Repair. Eur J Vasc Endovasc Surg. 2015 Jan;49(1):39-44.

[34] Perry RJT, Martin MJ, Eckert MJ, Sohn VY, Steele SR. Colonic ischemia complicating open vs endovascular abdominal aortic aneurysm repair. J Vasc Surg. 2008 Aug;48(2):272-277.

[35] Rayt HS, Bown MJ, Lambert KV, Fishwick NG, McCarthy MJ, London NJM, et al. Buttock claudication and erectile dysfunction after internal iliac artery embolization in patients prior to endovascular aortic aneurysm repair. Cardiovasc Intervent Radiol. 2008 Aug;31(4):728-734.

[36] Saratzis A, Melas N, Mahmood A, Sarafidis P. Incidence of Acute Kidney Injury (AKI) after Endovascular Abdominal Aortic Aneurysm Repair (EVAR) and Impact on Outcome. Eur J Vasc Endovasc Surg. 2015 May;49(5):534-540.

[37] Giles KA, Pomposelli F, Hamdan A, Wyers M, Jhaveri A, Schermerhorn ML. Decrease in total aneurysm-related deaths in the era of endovascular aneurysm repair. J Vasc Surg. 2009 Mar;49(3):543-550; discussion 550-551.

[38] Dillavou ED, Muluk SC, Makaroun MS. Improving

aneurysm-related outcomes: nationwide benefits of endovascular repair. J Vasc Surg. 2006 Mar;43(3):446-451; discussion 451-452.

[39] Greenberg RK, Sternbergh WC, Makaroun M, Ohki T, Chuter T, Bharadwaj P, et al. Intermediate results of a United States multicenter trial of fenestrated endograft repair for juxtarenal abdominal aortic aneurysms. J Vasc Surg. 2009 Oct;50(4):730-737.e1.

[40] Ricotta JJ, Oderich GS. Fenestrated and branched stent grafts. Perspect Vasc Surg Endovasc Ther. 2008 Jun;20(2):174-187; discussion 188-189.

[41] Schanzer A, Greenberg RK, Hevelone N, Robinson WP, Eslami MH, Goldberg RJ, et al. Predictors of abdominal aortic aneurysm sac enlargement after endovascular repair. Circulation. 2011 Jun 21;123(24):2848-2855.

[42] Moulakakis KG, Dalainas I, Mylonas S, Giannakopoulos TG, Avgerinos ED, Liapis CD. Conversion to open repair after endografting for abdominal aortic aneurysm: a review of causes, incidence, results, and surgical techniques of reconstruction. J Endovasc Ther. 2010 Dec;17(6):694-702.

[43] Peppelenbosch N, Buth J, Harris PL, van Marrewijk C, Fransen G, EUROSTAR Collaborators. Diameter of abdominal aortic aneurysm and outcome of endovascular aneurysm repair: does size matter? A report from EUROSTAR. J Vasc Surg. 2004 Feb;39(2):288-297.

[44] Howell M, Villareal R, Krajcer Z. Percutaneous access and closure of femoral artery access sites associated with endoluminal repair of abdominal aortic aneurysms. J Endovasc Ther. 2001 Feb;8(1):68-74.

[45] Torsello GB, Kasprzak B, Klenk E, Tessarek J, Osada N, Torsello GF. Endovascular suture versus cutdown for endovascular aneurysm repair: a prospective randomized pilot study. J Vasc Surg. 2003 Jul;38(1):78-82.

[46] Gimzewska M, Jackson AI, Yeoh SE, Clarke M. Totally percutaneous versus surgical cut-down femoral artery access for elective bifurcated abdominal endovascular aneurysm repair. Cochrane Database Syst Rev. 2017 Feb 21;2:CD010185.

[47] Ultee KHJ, Soden PA, Zettervall SL, Darling J, Verhagen HJM, Schermerhorn ML. Conversion from endovascular to open abdominal aortic aneurysm repair. J Vasc Surg. 2016 Jul;64(1):76-82.

[48] Phade SV, Keldahl ML, Morasch MD, Rodriguez HE, Pearce WH, Kibbe MR, et al. Late abdominal aortic endograft explants: indications and outcomes. Surgery. 2011 Oct;150(4):788-795.

[49] Brewster DC, Jones JE, Chung TK, Lamuraglia GM, Kwolek CJ, Watkins MT, et al. Long-term outcomes after endovascular abdominal aortic aneurysm repair: the first decade. Ann Surg. 2006 Sep;244(3):426-438.

[50] Brinster CJ, Fairman RM, Woo EY, Wang GJ, Carpenter JP, Jackson BM. Late open conversion and explantation of abdominal aortic stent grafts. J Vasc Surg. 2011 Jul;54(1):42-46.

[51] Mehta M, Veith FJ, Lipsitz EC, Ohki T, Russwurm G, Cayne NS, et al. Is elevated creatinine level a contraindication to endovascular aneurysm repair? J Vasc Surg. 2004 Jan;39(1):118-123.

[52] Preventza O, Wheatley GH, Ramaiah VG, Rodriguez-Lopez JA, Williams J, Olsen D, et al. Management of endoleaks associated with endovascular treatment of descending thoracic aortic diseases. J Vasc Surg. 2008 Jul;48(1):69-73.

[53] Blankensteijn JD, de Jong SECA, Prinssen M, van der Ham AC, Buth J, van Sterkenburg SMM, et al. Two-year outcomes after conventional or endovascular repair of abdominal aortic aneurysms. N Engl J Med. 2005 Jun 9;352(23):2398-2405.

[54] Feezor RJ, Huber TS, Martin TD, Beaver TM, Hess PJ, Klodell CT, et al. Perioperative differences between endovascular repair of thoracic and abdominal aortic diseases. J Vasc Surg. 2007 Jan;45(1):86-89.

[55] Gargiulo M, Gallitto E, Wattez H, Verzini F, Bianchini Massoni C, Loschi D, et al. Outcomes of endovascular aneurysm repair performed in abdominal aortic aneurysms with large infrarenal necks. J Vasc Surg. 2017 Oct;66(4):1065-1072.

[56] Oliveira NFG, Bastos Gonçalves FM, Van Rijn MJ, de Ruiter Q, Hoeks S, de Vries J-PPM, et al. Standard endovascular aneurysm repair in patients with wide infrarenal aneurysm necks is associated with increased risk of adverse events. J Vasc Surg. 2017 Jun;65(6):1608-1616.

[57] Umscheid T, Stelter WJ. Time-related alterations in shape, position, and structure of self-expanding, modular aortic stent-grafts: a 4-year single-center follow-up. J Endovasc Surg. 1999 Feb;6(1):17-32.

[58] England A, Butterfield JS, Jones N, McCollum CN, Nasim A, Welch M, et al. Device migration after endovascular abdominal aortic aneurysm repair: experience with a talent stent-graft. J Vasc Interv Radiol. 2004 Dec;15(12):1399-1405.

[59] de la Motte L, Kehlet H, Vogt K, Nielsen CH, Groenvall JB, Nielsen HB, et al. Preoperative methylprednisolone enhances recovery after endovascular aortic repair: a randomized, double-blind, placebo-controlled clinical trial. Ann Surg. 2014 Sep;260(3):540-548; discussion 548-549.

[60] Chaikof EL, Dalman RL, Eskandari MK, Jackson BM, Lee WA, Mansour MA, et al. The Society for Vascular Surgery practice guidelines on the care of patients with an abdominal aortic aneurysm. J Vasc Surg. 2018 Jan;67(1):2-77.e2.

[61] Pennell RC, Hollier LH, Lie JT, Bernatz PE, Joyce JW, Pairolero PC, et al. Inflammatory abdominal aortic aneurysms: a thirty-year review. J Vasc Surg. 1985 Nov;2(6):859-869.

[62] Bajardi G, Pecoraro F, Mirabella D, Bellisi MG. Inflammatory abdominal aortic aneurysm (IAAA). Ann Ital Chir. 2009 Jun;80(3):171-176.

[63] Paravastu SCV, Ghosh J, Murray D, Farquharson FG, Serracino-Inglott F, Walker MG. A systematic review of open versus endovascular repair of inflammatory abdominal aortic aneurysms. Eur J Vasc Endovasc Surg. 2009 Sep;38(3):291-297.

[64] Nakajima T, Kawazoe K, Komoda K, Sasaki T, Ohsawa S, Kamada T. Midline retroperitoneal versus midline transperitoneal approach for abdominal aortic aneurysm repair. J Vasc Surg. 2000 Aug;32(2):219-223.

[65] Endo M, Kobayashi K, Tsubota M, Seki M, Sato H, Noto T, et al. Advantages of using the midline incision right retroperitoneal approach for abdominal aortic aneurysm repair. Surg Today. 1996;26(1):1-4.

[66] Fassiadis N, Roidl M, Hennig M, South LM, Andrews SM. Randomized clinical trial of vertical or transverse laparotomy for abdominal aortic aneurysm repair. Br J Surg. 2005 Oct;92(10):1208-1211.

[67] Kawaharada N, Morishita K, Fukada J, Yamada A, Muraki S,

Hachiro Y, et al. Minilaparotomy abdominal aortic aneurysm repair versus the retroperitoneal approach and standard open surgery. Surg Today. 2004;34(10):837-841.

[68] Edwards JM, Teefey SA, Zierler RE, Kohler TR. Intraabdominal paraanastomotic aneurysms after aortic bypass grafting. J Vasc Surg. 1992 Feb;15(2):344-350; discussion 351-353.

[69] Coscas R, Greenberg RK, Mastracci TM, Eagleton M, Kang WC, Morales C, et al. Associated factors, timing, and technical aspects of late failure following open surgical aneurysm repairs. J Vasc Surg. 2010 Aug;52(2):272-281.

[70] Kadakol AK, Nypaver TJ, Lin JC, Weaver MR, Karam JL, Reddy DJ, et al. Frequency, risk factors, and management of perigraft seroma after open abdominal aortic aneurysm repair. J Vasc Surg. 2011 Sep;54(3):637-643.

[71] Djavani Gidlund K, Wanhainen A, Björck M. Intra-abdominal hypertension and abdominal compartment syndrome after endovascular repair of ruptured abdominal aortic aneurysm. Eur J Vasc Endovasc Surg. 2011 Jun;41(6):742-747.

[72] Capoccia L, Speziale F, Menna D, Esposito A, Sirignano P, Rizzo AR, et al. Preliminary Results from a National Enquiry of Infection in Abdominal Aortic Endovascular Repair (Registry of Infection in EVAR--R.I.EVAR). Ann Vasc Surg. 2016 Jan;30:198-204.

[73] Cernohorsky P, Reijnen MMPJ, Tielliu IFJ, van Sterkenburg SMM, van den Dungen JJAM, Zeebregts CJ. The relevance of aortic endograft prosthetic infection. J Vasc Surg. 2011 Aug;54(2):327-333.

[74] Ducasse E, Calisti A, Speziale F, Rizzo L, Misuraca M, Fiorani P. Aortoiliac stent graft infection: current problems and management. Ann Vasc Surg. 2004 Sep;18(5):521-526.

[75] O'Connor S, Andrew P, Batt M, Becquemin JP. A systematic review and meta-analysis of treatments for aortic graft infection. J Vasc Surg. 2006 Jul;44(1):38-45.

[76] Heyer KS, Modi P, Morasch MD, Matsumura JS, Kibbe MR, Pearce WH, et al. Secondary infections of thoracic and abdominal aortic endografts. J Vasc Interv Radiol. 2009 Feb;20(2):173-179.

[77] Grass F, Deglise S, Corpataux J-M, Saucy F. In situ aortobiiliac reconstruction of infected aneurysm using a single superficial femoral vein. Vasc Endovascular Surg. 2013 Jul;47(5):390-393.

[78] Dorweiler B, Neufang A, Schmiedt W, Oelert H. Autogenous reconstruction of infected arterial prosthetic grafts utilizing the superficial femoral vein. Thorac Cardiovasc Surg. 2001 Apr;49(2):107-111.

[79] Vogel TR, Symons R, Flum DR. The incidence and factors associated with graft infection after aortic aneurysm repair. J Vasc Surg. 2008 Feb;47(2):264-269.

[80] Orandi BJ, Dimick JB, Deeb GM, Patel HJ, Upchurch GR. A population-based analysis of endovascular versus open thoracic aortic aneurysm repair. J Vasc Surg. 2009 May;49(5):1112-1116.

[81] Milewicz DM, Dietz HC, Miller DC. Treatment of aortic disease in patients with Marfan syndrome. Circulation. 2005 Mar 22;111(11):e150–e157.

[82] Pepin M, Schwarze U, Superti-Furga A, Byers PH. Clinical and genetic features of Ehlers-Danlos syndrome type IV, the vascular type. N Engl J Med. 2000 Mar 9;342(10):673-680.

[83] Booher AM, Eagle KA. Diagnosis and management issues in thoracic aortic aneurysm. Am Heart J. 2011 Jul;162(1):38-46.e1.

[84] Patterson BO, Holt PJ, Nienaber C, Fairman RM, Heijmen RH, Thompson MM. Management of the left subclavian artery and neurologic complications after thoracic endovascular aortic repair. J Vasc Surg. 2014 Dec;60(6):1491-1497.e1.

[85] Klocker J, Koell A, Erlmeier M, Goebel G, Jaschke W, Fraedrich G. Ischemia and functional status of the left arm and quality of life after left subclavian artery coverage during stent grafting of thoracic aortic diseases. J Vasc Surg. 2014 Jul;60(1):64-69.

[86] Maldonado TS, Dexter D, Rockman CB, Veith FJ, Garg K, Arko F, et al. Left subclavian artery coverage during thoracic endovascular aortic aneurysm repair does not mandate revascularization. J Vasc Surg. 2013 Jan;57(1):116-124.

[87] Riesenman PJ, Farber MA, Mendes RR, Marston WA, Fulton JJ, Keagy BA. Coverage of the left subclavian artery during thoracic endovascular aortic repair. J Vasc Surg. 2007 Jan;45(1):90-94; discussion 94-95.

[88] Simonte G, Parlani G, Farchioni L, Isernia G, Cieri E, Lenti M, et al. Lesson Learned with the Use of Iliac Branch Devices: Single Centre 10 Year Experience in 157 Consecutive Procedures. Eur J Vasc Endovasc Surg. 2017 Jul;54(1):95-103.

[89] O'Callaghan A, Mastracci TM, Greenberg RK, Eagleton MJ, Bena J, Kuramochi Y. Outcomes for supra-aortic branch vessel stenting in the treatment of thoracic aortic disease. J Vasc Surg. 2014 Oct;60(4):914-920.

[90] Leon LR, Mills JL, Jordan W, Morasch MM, Kovacs M, Becker GJ, et al. The risks of celiac artery coverage during endoluminal repair of thoracic and thoracoabdominal aortic aneurysms. Vasc Endovascular Surg. 2009 Mar;43(1):51-60.

[91] Najibi S, Terramani TT, Weiss VJ, Mac Donald MJ, Lin PH, Redd DC, et al. Endoluminal versus open treatment of descending thoracic aortic aneurysms. J Vasc Surg. 2002 Oct;36(4):732-737.

[92] Cheung AT. An evolving role of anesthesiologists in the management of thoracic aortic diseases. Anesth Analg. 2010 Aug;111(2):259-260.

[93] Acher CW, Wynn M. A modern theory of paraplegia in the treatment of aneurysms of the thoracoabdominal aorta: An analysis of technique specific observed/expected ratios for paralysis. J Vasc Surg. 2009 May;49(5):1117-1124; discussion 1124.

[94] Eggebrecht H, Thompson M, Rousseau H, Czerny M, Lönn L, Mehta RH, et al. Retrograde ascending aortic dissection during or after thoracic aortic stent graft placement: insight from the European registry on endovascular aortic repair complications. Circulation. 2009 Sep 15;120(11 Suppl):S276–S281.

[95] Connolly JE. Hume Memorial lecture. Prevention of spinal cord complications in aortic surgery. Am J Surg. 1998 Aug;176(2):92-101.

[96] Czerny M, Eggebrecht H, Sodeck G, Verzini F, Cao P, Maritati G, et al. Mechanisms of symptomatic spinal cord ischemia after TEVAR: insights from the European Registry of Endovascular Aortic Repair Complications (EuREC). J Endovasc Ther. 2012 Feb;19(1):37-43.

[97] Buth J, Harris PL, Hobo R, van Eps R, Cuypers P, Duijm L, et al. Neurologic complications associated with endovascular repair of thoracic aortic pathology: Incidence and risk factors. a study from the European Collaborators on Stent/Graft Techniques for Aortic Aneurysm Repair (EUROSTAR) registry. J Vasc Surg. 2007 Dec;46(6):1103-1110; discussion 1110-1111.

[98] Greenberg RK, Lu Q, Roselli EE, Svensson LG, Moon MC, Hernandez AV, et al. Contemporary analysis of descending thoracic and thoracoabdominal aneurysm repair: a comparison of endovascular and open techniques. Circulation. 2008 Aug 19;118(8):808-817.

[99] Zoli S, Roder F, Etz CD, Brenner RM, Bodian CA, Lin H-M, et al. Predicting the risk of paraplegia after thoracic and thoracoabdominal aneurysm repair. Ann Thorac Surg. 2010 Oct;90(4):1237-1244; discussion 1245.

[100] Berg P, Kaufmann D, van Marrewijk CJ, Buth J. Spinal cord ischaemia after stent-graft treatment for infra-renal abdominal aortic aneurysms. Analysis of the Eurostar database. Eur J Vasc Endovasc Surg. 2001 Oct;22(4):342-347.

[101] Takayama H, Borger MA. Preventing spinal cord injury during thoracic aortic surgery: simpler than we thought? J Thorac Cardiovasc Surg. 2015 Jan;149(1):366-368.

[102] Di Luozzo G. Visceral and spinal cord protection during thoracoabdominal aortic aneurysm repair: clinical and laboratory update. J Thorac Cardiovasc Surg. 2013 Mar;145(3 Suppl):S135–S138.

[103] Svensson LG, Kouchoukos NT, Miller DC, Bavaria JE, Coselli JS, Curi MA, et al. Expert consensus document on the treatment of descending thoracic aortic disease using endovascular stent-grafts. Ann Thorac Surg. 2008 Jan;85(1 Suppl):S1-41.

[104] Vaddineni SK, Taylor SM, Patterson MA, Jordan WD. Outcome after celiac artery coverage during endovascular thoracic aortic aneurysm repair: preliminary results. J Vasc Surg. 2007 Mar;45(3):467-471.

[105] Nordon IM, Karthikesalingam A, Hinchliffe RJ, Holt PJ, Loftus IM, Thompson MM. Secondary interventions following endovascular aneurysm repair (EVAR) and the enduring value of graft surveillance. Eur J Vasc Endovasc Surg. 2010 May;39(5):547-554.

[106] Perek B, Juszkat R, Kulesza J, Jemielity M. Stent grafts separation 6 years after endovascular repair of a thoracic aortic aneurysm. J Vasc Interv Radiol. 2014 Oct;25(10):1650-1652.

[107] Shukla AJ, Jeyabalan G, Cho J-S. Late collapse of a thoracic endoprosthesis. J Vasc Surg. 2011 Mar;53(3):798-801.

[108] Matsumura JS, Cambria RP, Dake MD, Moore RD, Svensson LG, Snyder S, et al. International controlled clinical trial of thoracic endovascular aneurysm repair with the Zenith TX2 endovascular graft: 1-year results. J Vasc Surg. 2008 Feb;47(2):247-257; discussion 257.

[109] Makaroun MS, Dillavou ED, Wheatley GH, Cambria RP, Gore TAG Investigators. Five-year results of endovascular treatment with the Gore TAG device compared with open repair of thoracic aortic aneurysms. J Vasc Surg. 2008 May;47(5):912-918.

[110] Scali ST, Beck AW, Butler K, Feezor RJ, Martin TD, Hess PJ, et al. Pathology-specific secondary aortic interventions after thoracic endovascular aortic repair. J Vasc Surg. 2014 Mar;59(3):599-607.

[111] Szeto WY, Desai ND, Moeller P, Moser GW, Woo EY, Fairman RM, et al. Reintervention for endograft failures after thoracic endovascular aortic repair. J Thorac Cardiovasc Surg. 2013 Mar;145(3 Suppl):S165–S170.

[112] Dake MD, Miller DC, Mitchell RS, Semba CP, Moore KA, Sakai T. The "first generation" of endovascular stent-grafts for patients with aneurysms of the

descending thoracic aorta. J Thorac Cardiovasc Surg. 1998 Nov;116(5):689-703; discussion 703-704.

[113] Shapira OM, Aldea GS, Cutter SM, Fitzgerald CA, Lazar HL, Shemin RJ. Improved clinical outcomes after operation of the proximal aorta: a 10-year experience. Ann Thorac Surg. 1999 Apr;67(4):1030-1037.

[114] Achneck HE, Rizzo JA, Tranquilli M, Elefteriades JA. Safety of thoracic aortic surgery in the present era. Ann Thorac Surg. 2007 Oct;84(4):1180-1185; discussion 1185.

[115] Arabkhani B, Mookhoek A, Di Centa I, Lansac E, Bekkers JA, De Lind Van Wijngaarden R, et al. Reported Outcome After Valve-Sparing Aortic Root Replacement for Aortic Root Aneurysm: A Systematic Review and Meta-Analysis. Ann Thorac Surg. 2015 Sep;100(3):1126-1131.

[116] David TE, Feindel CM, Bos J. Repair of the aortic valve in patients with aortic insufficiency and aortic root aneurysm. J Thorac Cardiovasc Surg. 1995 Feb;109(2):345-351; discussion 351-352.

[117] Wheat MW, Wilson JR, Bartley TD. SUCCESSFUL REPLACEMENT OF THE ENTIRE ASCENDING AORTA AND AORTIC VALVE. JAMA. 1964 May 25;188:717-719.

Section 2

Special Situations

Chapter 6

Aortic Aneurysm in Pregnancy

Jennifer Chin and Marguerite Lisa Bartholomew

Abstract

Aortic aneurysms in pregnancy are rare but often fatal due to the natural physiologic changes of pregnancy and comorbidities specific to pregnancy, which increase the risk for aortic dissection and rupture. These physiologic changes are most pronounced in the third trimester and during the peripartum period, when approximately one third of dissections occur. In patients with known aortic aneurysms or conditions that make them prone to aortic aneurysms, preconception counseling can make pregnancy safer and more manageable. Aortic aneurysms diagnosed during pregnancy are usually due to underlying connective tissue diseases or aortopathies that have not been previously diagnosed. These women require multidisciplinary care including but not limited to obstetrics and gynecology, maternal fetal medicine, neonatology, cardiology, cardiothoracic surgery, cardiothoracic anesthesia, and genetics. Decisions include screening for dissection, when to proceed with surgical management, the best mode and timing for delivery, postpartum care, and contraception.

Keywords: aortic dissection, pregnancy, postpartum, delivery timing, contraception

1. Introduction

Aortic aneurysms in pregnancy are a rare but potentially fatal occurrence. The incidence in the general population is low at 2.6–3.5 per 100,000 person-years [1]. Women present with aortic aneurysms at an average age of 67 years, which is older than the average age of men presenting at 60 years. A significant index of suspicion is necessary to identify aortic aneurysms during pregnancy. Symptoms of aortic aneurysm or aortic dissection include significant chest pain that may or may not radiate to the back, dyspnea, syncope, and dysphagia. Chest x-ray (PA and lateral) should not be withheld for pregnant women with such symptoms. Although the cardiac silhouette may appear mildly enlarged on chest x-ray during pregnancy, persistent symptoms with or without a widened mediastinum should be evaluated with further imaging. In any patient, the highest morbidity and mortality results from an aortic dissection. **Table 1** shows types of aortic dissections, their description, and their associated mortality rates.

The highest mortality risk is a Stanford type A acute dissection, which describes an intimal tear involving the ascending aorta allowing blood to flow into the medial layer, which can ultimately culminate in aortic rupture leading to ischemia, tamponade, aortic regurgitation, or stroke. Stanford type A dissections typically present with a pulse deficit, systolic blood pressure limb differential of over 20 mmHg, focal neurologic deficits, or syncope [2]. Stanford type B dissections, which involve the descending aorta, have a lower mortality rate of 10% after 30 days. These are usually managed medically with strict blood pressure control as opposed to type A dissections, which typically require surgical management [2].

IntechOpen

Type of Dissection	Description	Mortality
Stanford type A	Involves ascending aorta	40%
Stanford type B	Involves descending aorta	10%

Table 1.
Types of aortic dissections and associated mortality rates [1].

Risk factors for aortic aneurysms and resulting aortic dissections vary depending on age. For older women in the general population, hypertension and atherosclerosis contribute to the development of aortic aneurysms and aortic dissections. In contrast, aortic aneurysms in reproductive aged women usually occur in the setting of an underlying connective tissue or genetic disorder, such as Marfan's disease, Ehlers-Danlos syndrome, Turner's syndrome, or Loeys-Dietz syndrome, or an underlying aortopathy, such as bicuspid aorta, coarctation of the aorta, familial thoracic aortic dissection syndrome, or aneurysm-osteoarthitis. Among women less than 40 years old with aortic aneurysms, pregnancy has been shown to increase the risk of dissection by up to 25 fold [1]. Fortunately, the incidence of aortic aneurysm in pregnancy is low at 0.05 per 100,000 person-years; however, maternal mortality is high and ranges from 21–53% [3]. Aortic dissections in pregnancy account for 0.1–0.4% of all dissections and represent 0.0004% of all pregnancies [4].

Due to the rare occurrence of aortic aneurysm and dissection in pregnancy, management is largely based on case series and expert opinion. Treatment is nuanced and complex often due to perceived conflicting priorities of maternal and fetal health. The family's wellbeing is absolutely dependent on maternal survival and long-term health so these are not actually separate priorities. This chapter will review the unique physiology and risk factors for aortic dissection in pregnant women with aortic aneurysms, optimal management of known aortic aneurysms in reproductive aged women prior to pregnancy, best practice guidelines for aortic aneurysms during pregnancy, mode and timing of delivery of the pregnancy, and recommendations for postpartum care including prevention of or planning for another high-risk pregnancy.

2. Aortic aneurysm and dissection in pregnancy

2.1 Physiology of pregnancy in aortic aneurysms

Aortic aneurysms in pregnancy have a much higher risk of progression to aortic dissection and rupture than aortic aneurysms in the general population. This difference is incompletely understood, but can be mostly explained by physiologic, specifically vascular, changes unique to pregnancy, as well as underlying connective tissue or genetic disorders that predispose reproductive aged women to aortic aneurysms. The clinical features of these diseases are often exacerbated in pregnancy and increase the morbidity and mortality of aortic aneurysms in pregnancy and the pregnancies themselves.

2.1.1 Vascular changes of pregnancy

During pregnancy, specific physiologic changes occur to support the fetus and prepare for childbirth. Cardiovascular changes begin in the first trimester and peak in the third trimester and peripartum period, starting at 28 weeks of gestation up until 4 weeks after delivery. The vascular changes of pregnancy can negatively impact the progression of an aortic aneurysm and significantly contribute to the increased risk of aortic dissection in aortic aneurysm in pregnancy. Some of these changes include increased cardiac output, heart rate, circulating volume, and left ventricular mass, all of which increase the risk of aortic dissection and rupture [1]. Estrogen and progesterone, both hormones that significantly increase in pregnancy, have been proven to change the microstructure of the aortic media and intima layers, causing fragmentation of reticulum fibers and loss of corrugation of elastic fibers [4]. This weakening of the vessel walls further contributes to the increased risk of aortic dissection and rupture. Some hypothesize that the gravid uterus, as it increases in size, compresses the aorta and thus increases the aortic outflow resistance, also increasing the risk of aortic dissection [1]. All of these vascular changes are most pronounced in the third trimester, when 50% of aortic dissections occur, and during the peripartum period, 4 weeks before and 4 weeks after delivery, when 33% of aortic dissections occur [2]. Certain conditions specific to pregnancy, such as pre-eclampsia, which causes vasoconstriction and sudden severe elevation of blood pressures, significantly increases the risk for aortic dissection and further complicates management.

2.1.2 Connective tissue and genetic disorders in pregnancy

There are several connective tissue and genetic disorders that predispose reproductive aged women to aortic aneurysms and have serious implications during pregnancy, both on the progression to aortic dissection and rupture as well as the pregnancy itself. While not an exhaustive list, the connective tissue and genetic disorders that will be discussed in this section include Marfan syndrome, Ehlers-Danlos syndrome, Loeys-Dietz syndrome, and Turner syndrome.

Marfan syndrome is an autosomal dominant connective tissue disorder that affects approximately 3 in 10,000 people [3]. Among pregnant women with aortic aneurysms, Marfan syndrome causes approximately half of aortic dissections [1]. It is characterized by musculoskeletal abnormalities including pectus excavatum, ocular abnormalities, cardiovascular abnormalities including aortic aneurysm and dissection, pulmonary abnormalities including spontaneous pneumothorax, skin abnormalities including stretch marks, and dura abnormalities including lumbosacral dural ectasia [5]. In the past, life expectancy was extremely limited, usually due to cardiovascular complications related to the disease; however, with current medical and surgical therapy, life expectancy can extend into the 70s. Diagnosis of Marfan syndrome can be made clinically based on criteria within different organ systems based on positive or negative family history. In the absence of family history, 2 major criteria from 2 different organ systems and 1 other major or minor criteria from another organ system must be met. In the presence of family history, only 1 major criterion and 1 major or minor criterion from a different organ system is necessary for diagnosis. Diagnosis can be confirmed by genetic testing, which will show a mutation on the fibrillin gene on chromosome 15.

During pregnancy, women with Marfan disease incur a high risk of morbidity and mortality due to the possibility of aortic dissection. This risk is particularly pronounced when aortic root dilation is over 4 cm. When the aortic root dilation is less than 4 cm, the risk of dissection is 1%; when the aortic root dilation is over 4 cm, the risk of dissection increases to 10%. Additionally, when aortic root dilation is over 4–4.5 cm, pregnant women will likely experience an accelerated rate of aortic root growth as compared to nonpregnant women [5]. In addition to maternal cardiovascular risk, there is likely an increased risk of obstetric and postpartum complications including a higher rate of preterm labor, preterm premature rupture of membranes, maternal urinary incontinence, and pelvic organ prolapse postpartum.

In nonpregnant patients, beta-blockers significantly slow the growth of the aortic root and decrease the risk of aortic dissection. There is some concern about the use of these medications in pregnancy due to possible adverse effects for the fetus including intrauterine growth restriction and fetal bradycardia. The risk benefit ratio supports the use of betablockers for treatment of aortic aneurysm during pregnancy. Selective beta-1 receptor blockers, such as metoprolol, are usually chosen due to a decreased risk of intrauterine growth restriction [5].

Several medications commonly used in obstetrics require careful use in pregnant women with Marfan syndrome. In cases of threatened preterm labor, tocolytics such as magnesium sulfate and calcium channel blockers can be used without significant adverse events. However, beta-adrenergic agonists, such as terbutaline, may increase the risk for tachycardia and arrhythmias and thus should be used with extreme caution. Additionally, indomethacin, commonly used for tocolysis in threatened preterm labor less than 32 weeks of gestation, can cause fluid retention, which may increase the risk for aortic dissection, and thus should also be used with extreme caution [5].

Ehlers-Danlos syndrome, less common than Marfan syndrome, occurs in approximately 1 in 5000 people. There are 6 different types of Ehlers-Danlos syndrome, which generally causes hypermobility of the joints, poor wound healing, tissue fragility, and hyperelastic skin [3]. The most severe type of Ehlers-Danlos syndrome and the most dangerous during pregnancy is the vascular type of disease. While hypermobility of the joints and hyperelasticity of the skin are less common in this type of disease, there is a significantly increased risk of aortic dissection, which is often not preceded by aortic dilation [3]. Due to tissue fragility, pregnant women with Ehlers-Danlos syndrome vascular type also have an increased risk of peripartum mortality up to 12% due to the risk of arterial or uterine rupture and hemorrhage [3].

Loeys-Dietz syndrome is a connective tissue disorder caused by mutation of the genes TGFBR1 or TGFBR2. Loeys-Dietz syndrome shares many characteristics with Marfan syndrome and Ehlers-Danlos syndrome vascular type. The disease is characterized by pectus excavatum, joint hypermobility, arterial tortuosity, hypertelorism, and bifid uvula [3]. Life expectancy for women with Loeys-Dietz syndrome is short with a mean age of death at 26 years, usually due to vascular complications. Similar to Marfan syndrome and Ehlers-Danlos syndrome vascular type, tissue fragility contributes to an increased risk of aortic dissection and uterine rupture, conferring significant morbidity and mortality in pregnancy.

Turner syndrome is a genetic disorder caused by complete or partial loss of one of the X chromosomes in a female. It occurs in approximately 1 in 2000 female births and is characterized by short stature, delayed puberty, premature ovarian failure, learning disabilities, bicuspid aortic valve, coarctation of the aorta, and aortic arch abnormalities [3]. Due to the high rate of aortopathy in women with Turner syndrome, the risk of aortic dissection in pregnancy is significantly elevated over the general population. While most women with Turner syndrome experience infertility due to premature ovarian failure, women with mosaic Turner syndrome may be fertile and thus capable of pregnancy. The risk of death from acute aortic dissection among pregnant women with Turner syndrome is 2%, and thus pregnancy is not recommended if a cardiac anomaly is present [3].

While knowledge of these connective tissue and genetic disorders may aid in diagnosis, aortic dissection may still occur in the absence of known risk factors and thus should remain on the differential for any pregnant woman who presents with chest pain radiating to her back.

2.2 Management prior to conception

Screening for aortic aneurysm should ideally be performed prior to conception in at-risk women. At-risk women include reproductive aged women with a personal or family history of aortic aneurysm or dissection in the past, known connective tissue or genetic disorder predisposing them to aortic aneurysm, known aortopathy, congenital heart disease, previous cardiac surgery, or significant trauma [4].

Any female with known aortic disease should receive proper family planning and contraceptive counseling as soon as and ideally before they are able to become pregnant. Important aspects of counseling include the significant risk to maternal health and the heritable nature of many underlying diseases that cause aortic aneurysm and dissection. After careful review of a woman's individual risk or based on a woman's family planning desires, surrogacy and adoption may be the safest route for parenthood. Women should be aware that deciding to become pregnant can have serious consequences to their own health.

Baseline workup includes referral to and establishment of care with a cardiologist if not already done, echocardiography, electrocardiogram, and genetic consultation if necessary. Routine medications must be reviewed to make sure they are not teratogenic as many patients are stable on warfarin, ACE inhibitors, and ARBs, all of which carry significant fetal risk with exposure in utero [4].

Among women with Marfan syndrome, elective surgery is generally recommended prior to conception when the baseline aortic root dilation is greater than 4.7 cm [5]. This is due to the maternal risk of death exceeding 10% [4]. Preconception care should include echocardiography to assess the proximal and distal aortic diameters and valvular and cardiac function. In women with significant ventricular enlargement, Holter monitoring is recommended to evaluate for arrhythmias.

Elective surgery should also be recommended prior to pregnancy in women with bicuspid aortic valve and aortic root dilation greater than 5 cm due to the maternal risk of death exceeding 10% [4]. Due to the high risk of aortic dissection, elective surgery prior to pregnancy is also recommended in the following situations: history of aortic valve surgery and aortic root dilation greater than 4.5 cm, Loeys-Dietz syndrome and aortic root dilation greater than 4.2 cm, any aortic root dilation greater than 5.5 cm regardless of underlying connective tissue disease, and symptomatic, traumatic, or syphilitic aneurysms [4].

Importantly, while physicians may make recommendations one way or another, women have autonomy over when and if they wish to become pregnant and thus care teams must be willing to support women's choices or refer to a team that can provide proper clinical care.

2.3 Management during pregnancy

After thorough counseling or if a woman desires pregnancy regardless of the risks, management of aortic aneurysm in pregnancy requires close follow up, multidisciplinary care, and a heightened index of suspicion for aortic dissection or need for surgical intervention.

2.3.1 Screening during pregnancy

After pregnancy is established, strict blood pressure control and serial imaging are necessary to evaluate the aortic root diameter. Depending on the baseline aortic root diameter and the underlying cause of aortic aneurysm, imaging can be obtained as frequently as every 4–8 weeks or as infrequently as every trimester throughout pregnancy and then postpartum [3]. Blood pressure control and heart rate control are recommended using beta-blockers to slow the growth of the aortic root and help prevent aortic dissection [5]. Prompt recognition of rapid growth of aortic aneurysm or aortic dissection is essential due to the high risk of progression to aortic rupture, maternal death, and poor fetal/neonatal outcomes. If the aortic root diameter is increasing too rapidly, surgery may be necessary during pregnancy to decrease the risk of aortic dissection.

2.3.2 Imaging during pregnancy

Physicians who are unfamiliar with imaging in pregnancy may worry about fetal risks with different imaging modalities. Echocardiogram is safe and sufficient to monitor stability or progression of known aortic aneurysm in pregnancy. CT or MRI should be used to evaluate the aortic arch or thoracic aorta if these areas are known or suspected to be involved during pregnancy. In the workup of aortic aneurysm, the benefit of an accurate diagnosis from a CT angiogram highly outweighs the radiation exposure risk for the maternal-fetal dyad and should not be withheld. The radiation exposure from a CT angiogram is 0.01–0.66 mGy, which is well below the threshold for fetal injury (50 mGy) [6].

In an acute situation, such as when an aortic dissection is suspected, it is important to select the correct and most accurate imaging modality. CT angiography imaging is considered the gold standard and accuracy of diagnosis of aortic dissection approaches 100% with the newest machines available at most hospitals [7]. Transesophageal echocardiography is usually sufficient for diagnosing dissection; however, studies have shown significant inter-observer variability. Magnetic resonance angiogram is able to properly evaluate left ventricular dysfunction; however, most imaging units refer acute patients to CT angiography due to the time sensitive nature of diagnosis of aortic dissection [8].

2.3.3 Surgery during pregnancy

When aortic aneurysm or aortic dissection occurs in pregnancy, management is largely based on case series and expert opinion. Withholding indicated surgery from a pregnant woman as a result of concern for teratogenesis, pregnancy loss, preterm birth, or litigation is unfounded, and may significantly contribute to both maternal and neonatal morbidity [9]. Recommendations for aortic aneurysm treatment and surgery triage are based on nonpregnant individuals. **Table 2** shows differing society guidelines for evidence-based timing of surgical intervention. In general, if the aortic root diameter exceeds 5 cm, rapid progression in size is noted, or there is aortic valve regurgitation, surgical intervention during pregnancy is recommended and the benefits absolutely outweigh the risks [3]. While there is no standardized definition of rapid progression, most agree that an increase of more than 3–5 mm is significant. Pregnant women with aortic aneurysms are more likely to have an underlying aortopathy, which should decrease thresholds for surgical repair as risk for aortic dissection, aortic rupture, and maternal death are increased. Preeclampsia also increases risk for dissection and rupture. Studies have also shown an increased risk of mortality for patients with shorter stature, independent of size of aneurysm, and thus some experts recommend basing clinical decisions on the maximal cross-sectional area, which is calculated by dividing the square centimeters of the maximal aortic root diameter by the patient's height in meters, rather than the absolute aortic root diameter. When this measurement is used, surgical intervention during pregnancy is recommended if the ratio is above 10 [4].

Society	Recommendation
Canadian society for vascular surgery	Aortic root diameter at or above 5 cm, less if growing faster than 10% per year
Japanese circulation society	Aortic root diameter at or above 6 cm, 5 cm if accompanied by pain
European society of cardiology	Aortic root diameter greater than 5.5 cm, less if there is an indication for surgery on the aortic valve to combine surgeries
American college of cardiology	Aortic root diameter at or above 5.5 cm, less if growing faster than 0.5 cm/year, 4-5 cm or maximal cross sectional area greater than 10 with aortopathy or bicuspid aortic valve

**Symptomatic patients or patients with aortic dissection require urgent surgical intervention regardless of aortic root diameter.*

Table 2.
Society guidelines for surgical intervention of asymptomatic thoracic aortic aneurysms [3, 10].*

Contrary to popular belief, cardiopulmonary bypass (CPB), which is necessary for cardiothoracic surgical intervention, is not strictly contraindicated during pregnancy. The optimal mode and timing of delivery in relation to cardiothoracic surgery is discussed in the next section, but for some women, continuing pregnancy during CPB may be considered if they have compelling surgical indications and a previable or extremely preterm fetus. During CPB, several modifications can improve the fetal mortality rate below 20%, including performing the procedure under normothermic conditions in the left lateral decubitus position to maintain placental perfusion and decrease the risk of uterine contractions and preterm labor, high pump flow rate over 2.5–2.7 $L/min^{-1}/m^{-2}$ to maintain placental perfusion, short CPB and aortic cross-clamp time, perfusion above 70 mmHg, and hematocrit over 28% [5, 11].

For some women, particularly in the late second or third trimester, cesarean delivery immediately before cardiothoracic surgical intervention is the preferred management option. A common misconception in this scenario is excessive uterine bleeding if CPB and full anticoagulation are performed soon after cesarean delivery. Post cesarean bleeding is controlled physiologically by myometrial contraction and a two-layer suture closure. Preventative and early detection strategies include leaving the laparotomy open during the cardiothoracic surgery to directly evaluate and manage any intra-abdominal bleeding, placement of a prophylactic intrauterine balloon to provide uterine tamponade, or active monitoring of vaginal bleeding with the use of Allen stirrups [5]. In a case series, twenty-one mothers who had CPB initiated immediately after cesarean delivery had an average blood loss of 800 mL. None had excessive bleeding requiring abdominal packing or hysterectomy, and none used the additional preventative strategies mentioned above [11].

2.3.4 Fetal diagnosis of Aortopathy

Genetic screening or testing of the fetus is recommended for autosomal dominant aortopathies due to the high risk of transmission in the offspring. This information can be used for delivery and neonatal care planning, such as what level of care is needed, or it can be used by parents to determine whether or not to continue this particular pregnancy. These conditions include but are not limited to Marfan syndrome, Ehlers-Danlos syndrome, and Loeys-Dietz syndrome. This can be accomplished by chorionic villus sampling or amniocentesis. Unfortunately, even after obtaining fetal or placental cells, diagnosis of Marfan syndrome in the fetus may be missed as there are hundreds of mutations that have been identified on the fibrillin 1 gene, and not all of them have been definitely linked to Marfan syndrome [7]. Fetal sonographic findings may assist in fetal diagnosis of Marfan syndrome, such as cardiomegaly, dilated ascending aorta, dilated pulmonary artery, or dysplastic atrioventricular valves [7].

2.4 Mode and timing of delivery

Optimal management for the health of the mother and fetus depends on the size of the aortic aneurysm, presence or absence of aortic dissection, presence of underlying aortopathy, fetal gestational age, and desires for the pregnancy. Multidisciplinary counseling and informed consent are essential and complicated. This section will review best practices for the mode of delivery, including assisted vaginal or cesarean, and timing of delivery in relation to cardiothoracic surgical repair.

2.4.1 Mode of delivery

In pregnant women with aortic aneurysms, the mode of delivery depends on the presence of aortopathy, size, and stability of the aortic aneurysm. Vaginal delivery is recommended for women with aortic root diameters less than 4 cm. Epidural for adequate analgesia to help maintain blood pressure and heart rate control is recommended. Among pregnant women with Marfan syndrome, dural ectasia, or dural sac dilation, should be ruled out prior to epidural placement as they may often be asymptomatic in up to 90% of patients with Marfan syndrome [7]. Strict blood pressure control with antihypertensive medications and an assisted second stage of labor with either vacuum or forceps is recommended to decrease the risk of dissection [3].

Cesarean delivery is recommended for women with an aortic root diameter over 4 cm, severe aortic valve regurgitation, significant progression of aortic aneurysm, or history of a previous dissection or repair [7]. Detailed planning and communication with anesthesia, cardiology, and cardiothoracic surgery are necessary regardless of the mode of delivery.

2.4.2 Timing of delivery

Prior to fetal viability, providers must have a discussion with women about the option of or recommendation for pregnancy termination. For example, Marfan syndrome and other aortopathies with an aortic root size greater than 4 cm is an indication for pregnancy termination due to the significant risk of maternal death if the pregnancy is continued. If cardiothoracic surgical repair is indicated before fetal viability, termination of pregnancy should be strongly considered due to the fetal loss rate of up to 33% and the increased potential for long term neurologic impairment after CPB [12]. The definition of fetal viability is nuanced and depends on the woman's personal beliefs, the accuracy of gestational age dating, a particular state's legislation, and institutional guidelines. The American College of Obstetricians and Gynecologists defines the periviable period as between 20 and 25 weeks of gestation. Deliveries under 20 weeks 0 days are defined as spontaneous abortions. With accurate gestational age dating, there is no survival of neonates delivered at 20 and 21 weeks. Although there have been significant advances in neonatal intensive care, individualized and evidence-based conversations about neonate survival and life without significant neurologic impairment are essential.

After fetal viability, the decision analysis shifts to decisions about CPB and cardiac surgery with the fetus remaining in utero or delivery of the fetus just before the cardiac surgery. Risks of prematurity include but are not limited to neonatal death, low birthweight, respiratory distress, and neuro-developmental disabilities. Before 32 weeks of gestation, maternal administration of intravenous magnesium sulfate is recommended for fetal neuroprotection to reduce the risk of cerebral palsy. Before 34 weeks of gestation, corticosteroids are recommended for fetal lung maturation [13]. While there is no consensus, most experts recommend cesarean delivery immediately followed by CPB starting at 28–32 weeks of gestation as it is thought that at this gestational age, the benefits of delivery without exposure to maternal CPB outweigh the risks of neonatal prematurity [4, 5]. Advances in neonatal intensive care have improved neonatal survival and a lower gestational age for delivery may be reasonable (above 25 weeks) if the patient chooses to avoid the fetal risk of CPB and accept the risks of prematurity.

Before approximately 25 weeks of gestation, surgical repair via CPB with a viable fetus in utero may be the best management plan. The obstetrician and patient must then decide whether to monitor the fetal heart rate during cardiac surgery and what actions should be taken in the event of nonreassuring fetal heart rate, such as perfusion adjustments, intrauterine resuscitation, or delivery. This discussion requires shared decision making and multidisciplinary planning [5]. If neither urgent cesarean delivery nor intrauterine resuscitation are available or desired, intraoperative fetal monitoring is not necessary and may cause more harm than benefit. At all time points throughout the surgery, maternal life should be prioritized as maternal cardiac arrest or severe hypoxemia will most certainly lead to fetal death or extreme fetal morbidity. After 20 weeks gestation during a maternal cardiac arrest, the uterus should be emptied by hysterotomy no later than 4–5 minutes after arrest to maximize venous return and efficacy of maternal resuscitation efforts. If the fetus is viable, delivery no later than 4–5 minutes after maternal cardiac arrest and resuscitation also results in good neonatal outcomes. Tocodynamometry, to monitor uterine contractions, is generally recommended intraoperatively (when feasible) and postoperatively. Preterm contractions are common during and after CPB and may or may not result in preterm labor [5].

2.5 Postpartum care

Equally as important as managing acute complications of aortic aneurysm in pregnancy is planning for or prevention of the next high-risk pregnancy. This section discusses optimization of care in the postpartum period after delivery and options for contraception should the patient desire prevention of another pregnancy.

2.5.1 Postpartum surveillance

The postpartum period represents a particularly vulnerable timeframe for women as many of them will lose insurance coverage, neglect to care for themselves due to focus on their newborn, and are recovering from their delivery and potentially cardiothoracic surgery as well. The physiologic changes of pregnancy do not immediately return to pre-pregnancy after delivery, and many of the cardiovascular changes persist beyond the traditional 6 week postpartum period, when most women's insurance companies will terminate their coverage. In a recent cohort-crossover study, researchers found that the risk of aortic dissection and rupture remain increased as compared to the general population as long as 1 year after delivery [14]. This elevated risk of morbidity and mortality emphasizes the need for careful coordination of postpartum care and surveillance, including regular follow up with cardiology and obstetrics and gynecology, careful maintenance of medication, and routine imaging and lab work.

2.5.2 Contraception

The postpartum period is a critical time to discuss contraception and plans for childbearing in the future. Unfortunately, due to the medical complexity of these patients and the effort required to coordinate care effectively, contraception is often forgotten in the care of the recently postpartum woman with an aortic aneurysm or aortic dissection during pregnancy. As mentioned earlier in this chapter, the discussion of family planning and contraception has ideally already occurred before or as soon as women with known aortic aneurysms are able to become pregnant. If this has not occurred, it is beneficial to discuss contraception during the prenatal course so that a plan is made for after delivery. If this has not occurred, this discussion can happen during the postpartum period. Primary care providers, cardiologists, and cardiothoracic surgeons may not be equipped to discuss the safest and most reliable contraceptive options with patients, and thus this discussion may be best suited for the obstetrician/gynecologist. Ideally, cardiologists and surgeons should become familiar with selective contraceptive methods (such as the progestin-only injectable) to provide short term so that women with cardiovascular disease do not conceive before seeing an obstetrician/gynecologist.

The Centers for Disease Control and Prevention developed the US Medical Eligibility Criteria (US MEC) for Contraceptive Use, which gives standardized recommendations for each type of contraceptive method in the setting of certain medical conditions [15]. In patients with complicated valvular heart disease, estrogen containing hormonal contraceptive methods are contraindicated due to the increased risk of heart attack and stroke. However, all other methods including the copper and levonorgestrel IUDs, the etonogestrel implant, the progestin-only injectable, and progestin-only pills, are considered safe and effective for these women. Contraceptive counseling should include discussion of a woman's priorities in different aspects of the contraceptive method, such as efficacy, side effects, patient autonomy, and future pregnancy plans.

3. Conclusion

Aortic aneurysm in pregnancy is a rare occurrence that leads to increased maternal, fetal, and neonatal morbidity and mortality. Specific changes to women's physiology and complications unique to pregnancy predispose pregnant women with aortic aneurysm to aortic dissection; therefore a high index of suspicion is lifesaving. Pregnant women with aneurysms are likely to have an underlying collagen disorder or aortopathy and are at even higher risk for aortic root diameter growth and progression to aortic dissection, rupture, and death. Such underlying conditions also increase the risk for poor obstetrical outcomes such as uterine rupture, premature delivery, and maternal hemorrhage. In women who are known to be at-risk for aortic aneurysm or aortic dissection, management and counseling prior to conception is essential and should include discussion of highly effective contraception, surrogacy, and adoption. Management of aortic aneurysm in pregnancy requires multidisciplinary care, imaging, and medication management. Indicated surgery should not be withheld simply because of the pregnancy or provider discomfort as absence of treatment results in worse outcomes. Decisions regarding surgery and mode and timing of delivery are nuanced, complicated, and require shared patient centered decision making, effective communication, and cooperation from multiple specialists in a tertiary care center. With careful planning, adequate facilities, and skilled providers, favorable outcomes for mother and baby are possible for patients who experience aortic aneurysm and dissection in pregnancy.

Acknowledgements

We gratefully acknowledge the Sharma Foundation for their funding of this chapter to allow open access publication for widespread dissemination of this chapter's information.

Conflict of interest

The authors declare no conflict of interest.

Author details

Jennifer Chin[1*] and Marguerite Lisa Bartholomew[2]

1 University of Washington, Seattle, WA, USA

2 University of Hawaii, Honolulu, HI, USA

*Address all correspondence to: jmyc@uw.edu

References

[1] Zhu JM, Ma WG, Peters S. Aortic dissection in pregnancy: management strategy and outcomes. Annals of Thoracic Surgery. 2017;103:1199-1206.

[2] Rajagopalan S, Nwazota N, Chandrasekhar S. Outcomes in pregnant women with acute aortic dissections. International Journal of Obstetric Anesthesia. 2014;23(4):348-356.

[3] vanHagen I, Roos J. Aortopathology and pregnancy. Best Practice and Research: Clinical Obstetrics and Gynecology. 2014;28(4):537-550.

[4] Smok D. Aortopathy in pregnancy. Seminars in Perinatology. 2014;38:295-303.

[5] Houston L, Sullivan S. Marfan syndrome and vascular dissections during pregnancy. Minerva gynecology. 2012;64(5):409-419.

[6] Guidelines for diagnostic imaging during pregnancy and lactation. Committee Opinion No. 723. American College of Obstetricians and Gynecologists. Obstet Gynecol 2017;130:e210-6.

[7] Hartnell G. Imaging of aortic aneurysms and dissection. Journal of Thoracic Imaging. 2001;16(1):35-46.

[8] Saliba E, Sia Y. The ascending aortic aneurysm: when to intervene? International Journal of Cardiology. 2015;6:91-100.

[9] Nonobstetric surgery during pregnancy. Committee Opinion No. 775. American College of Obstetricians and Gynecologists. Obstet Gynecol 2019;133:e285-6.

[10] Hiratzka L, Bakris G, Beckman J, et al. American College of Cardiology Foundation/American Heart Association Task Force on Practice Guidelines; American Association for Thoracic surgery; American College of Radiology; American Stroke Association; Society of Cardiovascular Anesthesiologists; Society for Cardiovascular Angiography and Interventions; Society of Interventional Radiology; Society of Thoracic Surgeons; Society for Vascular Medicine. 2010 ACCF/AHA/AATS/ACR/ASA/SCA/SCAI/SIR/STS/SVM Guidelines for the diagnosis and management of patients with thoracic aortic disease: Executive summary: A report of the American College of Cardiology Foundation/American Heart Association Task Force on Practice Guidelines, American Association for Thoracic Surgery, American College of Radiology, American Stroke Association, Society of Cardiovascular Anesthesiologists, Society for Cardiovascular Angiography and Interventions, Society of Interventional Radiology, Society of Thoracic Surgeons, and Society for Vascular Medicine. Anesthesia and Analgesia. 2010 Aug;111(2):279-315.

[11] John A, Gurley F, Schaff HJ. Cardiopulmonary bypass during pregnancy. Annals of Thoracic Surgery. 2011;91(4):1191-1196.

[12] Liu Y, Han F, Zhuang J. Cardiac operation under cardiopulmonary bypass during pregnancy. Journal of Cardiothoracic Surgery. 2020;15(1):92.

[13] Periviable birth. Obstetric Care Consensus No. 6. American College of Obstetricians and Gynecologists. Obstetrics and Gynecology. 2017;130:e187-199.

[14] Kamel H, Roman M, Pitcher A, Devereux R. Pregnancy and the risk of aortic dissection or rupture. Circulation. 2016;134(7):527-533.

[15] Curtis K, Tepper N, Jatlaoui T, et al. U.S. medical eligibility criteria for contraceptive use. 2016;65:1-104.